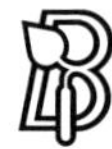

Milestones in Drug Therapy
MDT

Treatment of Psoriasis

Edited by Jeffrey M. Weinberg

Birkhäuser
Basel · Boston · Berlin

Editor
Jeffrey M. Weinberg
Department of Dermatology
St. Luke's-Roosevelt Hospital Center
1090 Amsterdam Avenue, Suite 11 D
New York, NY 10025
USA

Library of Congress Control Number: 2007936202

Bibliographic information published by Die Deutsche Bibliothek
Die Deutsche Bibliothek lists this publication in the Deutsche Nationalbibliografie; detailed bibliographic data is available in the internet at http://dnb.ddb.de

ISBN: 978-3-7643-7722-9 Birkhäuser Verlag AG, Basel – Boston – Berlin

Part of Springer Science+Business Media
Printed on acid-free paper produced from chlorine-free pulp. TFC ∞
Cover illustration: With the friendly permission by the American Society for Clinical Investigation
Printed in Germany

ISBN 978-3-7643-7722-9 e-ISBN 978-3-7643-7724-3

9 8 7 6 5 4 3 2 1 www. birkhauser.ch

Contents

List of contributors

Rahat S. Azfar, Department of Dermatology, University of Pennsylvania, 3600 Spruce St, 2 Maloney, Philadelphia, PA 19104, USA

Allison J. Brown, Department of Dermatology, Murdough Family Center for Psoriasis, University Hospitals Case Medical Center, 11100 Euclid Ave, Cleveland, OH 44106, USA

Paru R. Chaudhari, Mount Sinai School of Medicine, Department of Dermatology, 5 E 98th St 5th Floor, New York, NY 10029, USA; e-mail: paru.chaudhari@mssm.edu

Alissa Cowden, University of Pennsylvania, Philadelphia, PA 19104, USA

Neil J. Korman, Department of Dermatology, Murdough Family Center for Psoriasis, University Hospitals Case Medical Center, 11100 Euclid Ave, Cleveland, OH 44106, USA; e-mail: neil.korman@uhhospitals.org

Mark G. Lebwohl, Mount Sinai School of Medicine, Department of Dermatology, 5 E 98th St 5th Floor, New York, NY 10029, USA; e-mail: mark.lebwohl@mssm.edu

Marissa D. Newman, UMDNJ-Robert Wood Johnson Medical School New Jersey, New Jersey, 08902, USA; e-mail: marissa.newman@gmail.com

Edward M. Prodanovic, Department of Dermatology, Murdough Family Center for Psoriasis, University Hospitals Case Medical Center, 11100 Euclid Ave, Cleveland, OH 44106, USA

Maria R. Robinson, Department of Dermatology, Murdough Family Center for Psoriasis, University Hospitals Case Medical Center, Cleveland, OH 44106, USA

Sejal K. Shah, St. Luke's-Roosevelt Hospital Center, Department of Dermatology, 1090 Amsterdam Avenue, Suite 11D, New York, NY 10025, USA; e-mail: sejalshah151@yahoo.com

Amanda B. Sergay, Department of Dermatology, St. Luke's-Roosevelt Hospital Center and Beth Israel Medical Center, New York, NY, USA; e-mail: asergay@yahoo.com

Matthew Silvan, Department of Dermatology, St. Luke's-Roosevelt Hospital Center and Beth Israel Medical Center, New York, NY, USA

Dana K. Stern, Mount Sinai School of Medicine, Department of Dermatology, 5 E 98th St 5th Floor, New York, NY 10029, USA

Abby S. Van Voorhees, Psoriasis and Phototherapy Treatment Center, 2M44 Rhoads Pavilion, 3600 Spruce Street, Philadelphia, PA 19104, USA; e-mail: vanvoora@uphs.upenn.edu

Jeffrey M. Weinberg, Department of Dermatology, St. Luke's-Roosevelt Hospital Center and Beth Israel Medical Center, 1090 Amsterdam Avenue, Suite 11D, New York, NY 10025, USA; e-mail: jmw27@columbia.edu

Preface

Psoriasis is an inherited skin disease that has been diagnosed in 4.5 million adults in the US. About 10–30% of people with psoriasis also develop psoriatic arthritis, which causes pain, stiffness and swelling in and around the joints.

The past 25 years of research and clinical practice have revolutionized our understanding of the pathogenesis of psoriasis as the dysregulation of immunity triggered by environmental and genetic stimuli. Psoriasis was originally regarded as a primary disorder of epidermal hyperproliferation. However, experimental models and clinical results from immunomodulating therapies have refined this perspective in conceptualizing psoriasis as a genetically programmed pathologic interaction between resident skin cells, infiltrating immunocytes and a host of proinflammatory cytokines, chemokines and growth factors produced by these immunocytes.

The main focus of this volume will be the evolving paradigm of therapy for psoriasis. The first segment of the volume provides a background for the disease. The first two chapters will review the history of psoriasis and psoriasis therapy, and the pathophysiology of psoriasis. The third chapter provides a detailed clinical review of psoriasis and psoriatic arthritis.

The review of therapy begins in the next segment of the volume. Chapters 4 and 5 review the myriad of topical therapies available for psoriasis, and Chapter 6 discusses the spectrum of ultraviolet therapies and novel laser therapies for the treatment of this condition. Prior to the advent of biologic therapies, a number of oral therapies were the mainstay of systemic treatment for psoriasis. The efficacy and safety of these agents will be reviewed in Chapters 7 and 8.

Over the last few years, one of the major focuses in psoriasis research has been the development of biologic therapies for this disease. The aim of these therapies is to provide selective, immunologically directed intervention with fewer side effects than traditional therapies. Chapter 9 will review biologic therapy for psoriasis, providing an overview of infliximab, etanercept, adalimumab, efalizumab, and alefacept. Biologic and oral therapies in development will be discussed in Chapter 10.

Psoriasis-related quality of life is a broad term that aims to incorporate the physical, psychosocial, and economic implications of the disease, and their cumulative impact on the patient. The final chapter will address the important topic of quality of life issues in psoriasis.

The treatment of psoriasis is truly an evolving field. In the volume, an outstanding group of authors have provided the most recent clinical data, encompassing proper applications, efficacy, and safety. We hope that you will find the information useful in the scope of your research or practice. We urge you, however, to keep abreast of this field after reading this volume, as the flow of new information is constant.

Jeffrey M. Weinberg, MD New York, August 2007

Treatment of Psoriasis
Edited by J.M. Weinberg

Introduction: History of psoriasis and psoriasis therapy

Alissa Cowden and Abby S. Van Voorhees

University of Pennsylvania, Philadelphia, PA 19104, USA

Introduction

This chronicle of psoriasis begins in ancient times when psoriasis, leprosy, and other inflammatory skin disorders were thought to be the same condition. The identification of psoriasis as a distinct entity did not occur until the 19th century, when clinical descriptions distinguished it from other cutaneous disorders. Histopathologic descriptions in the 1960s and 1970s shed some light on the pathophysiology of psoriasis, but many aspects of the disease remain unknown to this day. As Bechet expressed, "Psoriasis is an antidote for dermatologists' ego" [1].

Given the lack of understanding of its pathophysiology, early psoriasis therapies were discovered serendipitously. Chance observations by early clinicians of psoriatic improvement in patients prescribed medications for other conditions led to advancements in therapy. As our understanding grew, this serendipity evolved into detailed targeting of specific immunological processes. These newly directed therapies clarified aspects of the pathophysiology and treatment of psoriasis and other immune-mediated diseases.

Ancient history: Lepra, psora, psoriasis

The roots of the identification of psoriasis lie in Ancient Greece. The Greeks, who pioneered the field of medicine, divided skin disease into the categories of *psora, lepra* and *leichen* [2]. *Psora* referred to itch, while *lepra* was derived from the Greek words *lopos* (the epidermis) and *lepo* (to scale) [3]. Hippocrates (460–377 BC) was one of the first authors to write descriptions of skin disorders. He utilized the word *lopoi* to describe the dry, scaly, disfiguring eruptions of psoriasis, leprosy, and other inflammatory skin disorders [4].

Similar to Hippocrates' works, the Old Testament also lumped together many cutaneous disorders. The biblical term *tsaraat,* or *zaraath,* described a range of skin conditions including leprosy and psoriasis. Lepers were often ostracized because they were considered divinely punished, and cruelty was imposed upon those who suffered from psoriasis and leprosy alike [5, 6].

Many historians credit the Roman thinker Celsus (ca. 25 BC–45 AD) with the first clinical description of papulosquamous diseases [1, 2, 5]. Celsus described impetigines and specified that the second species of impetigo was characterized by red skin covered with scales. This description suggested a type of papulosquamous disease, such as psoriasis [7].

Galen (133–200 AD) first utilized the term psoriasis, but his description was not consistent with the disorder that we now call psoriasis. He described psoriasis as a pruritic, scaly skin disease of the eyelids and scrotum. Although he used the term psoriasis, his description is now believed to most likely represent seborrheic dermatitis [4, 5, 8].

Indiscriminate grouping together of all inflammatory skin diseases led to stigmatization of patients with psoriasis. For centuries, patients with psoriasis received the same cruel handling as lepers. They were required to carry a bell or clapper to announce their approach, and had to wear a special dress. In addition, they could only touch or dine with others considered lepers. In 1313, Phillip the Fair of France ordered that they be burned at the stake [1].

Distinguishing psoriasis as a distinct entity

In 1809, Willan built on Celsus's description of papulosquamous conditions by detailing features of what we now know as psoriasis. However, he described modern psoriasis under the term lepra vulgaris, which perpetuated confusion of psoriasis and leprosy. Lepra vulgaris was described as enlarging, sharply marginated erythematous plaques with silvery-white scale that occurred most frequently on the knees, and were associated with nail pitting [8, 9].

For decades after Willan's description, some authors favored using the term psoriasis [1, 2, 10–12], while others chose the term lepra [9, 13]. Physicians lacked clarity regarding the word psoriasis and the ability to distinguish psoriasis from diseases with similar cutaneous manifestations.

Finally, Gibert and Hebra matched Willan's description with the term psoriasis, ending much confusion. Psoriasis was now finally acknowledged as a distinct disease, leading to improved perception of psoriatic patients.

In his books, Gibert (1797–1866) used the term psoriasis, recognized secondary syphilis as a contagious entity, and established pityriasis rosea as a clinical syndrome. Gibert's pivotal publications included thorough accounts that made important distinctions between papulosquamous diseases [5, 10, 14]. In 1841, shortly after Gibert's works, Hebra further distinguished the clinical picture of psoriasis from that of leprosy. Only 165 years ago, this differentiation set the stage for psoriatic patient's freedom from extreme persecution [15, 16]. The distinctions made by Gibert and Hebra were essential to accurately diagnosing patients and developing tailored therapies.

Advancements in the description of psoriasis

The 19th century identification of psoriasis as a separate entity ushered in a period of increasingly accurate descriptions of the disease. One of Hebra's students, Heinrich Auspitz (1835–1886), noted bleeding points upon removal of scale in patients with psoriasis. We now refer to this as the Auspitz sign [14, 17]. Along with the Auspitz sign, the Köbner reaction is a characteristic feature of psoriasis. In 1876, Köbner described the propensity of psoriatic lesions to arise in areas of prior trauma. Köbner's observation provided insight into the importance of the vascular compartment in the initiation of the psoriatic lesion [18]. Two decades later, in 1898, Munro described microabscesses of psoriasis that are now known as Munro's abscesses [17].

The start of the 20th Century ushered in further descriptions of psoriatic lesions. In 1910, Leo von Zumbusch first described generalized pustular psoriasis, or von Zumbusch disease [19]. Additional descriptions included Woronoff's 1926 description of a pale halo referred to as the 'Woronoff ring' encircling a plaque of psoriasis [20]. The portrayals of the Auspitz sign, Köbner's phenomenon, Munro's abscesses, pustular prosiasis, and the Woronoff ring allowed physicians to more confidently diagnose patients with psoriasis.

Understanding pathophysiology

In addition to clinical observations, histopathologic descriptions of psoriatic skin advanced understanding of the roles of epidermal hyperplasia and the immune system in psoriasis. Epidermal hyperplasia in psoriasis was first observed in 1963, when Van Scott noted a significant increase in mitoses of psoriatic epidermis [21]. Three years later, Van Scott and Weinstein noted that psoriatic basal cells rose to the stratum corneum in only two days, in contrast to their 12 day transit through normal epidermis [22].

Therapeutic discoveries and histopathologic observations linked the immune system with psoriasis. In 1951, Gubner treated rheumatoid arthritis with the folic acid antagonist aminopterin, and serendipitously noted clearing of the skin in patients with psoriasis [23]. At that time researchers did not understand the mechanism of action of folic acid antagonists in psoriasis treatment, but later understanding revealed that these medications modulated the immune system. Two decades after Gubner's report, Mueller prescribed cyclosporine to prevent rejection in transplant patients, and found improvement of lesions in patients with psoriasis [24]. Reports of psoriatic improvement provided by immunosuppressive drugs implicated the immune system in the pathogenesis of psoriasis. Histopathologic observations, that cellular infiltrates in psoriasis were composed primarily of T cells and macrophages, further highlighted the role of the immune system in psoriasis [25, 26].

In spite of these discoveries, much remains unknown about the pathogenesis of psoriasis and other immune-mediated diseases including arthritis and inflammatory bowel disease. Psoriasis serves as a model for immune-mediated diseases because the response to therapy can be readily seen [27].

History of treatment of psoriasis

The history of the treatment of psoriasis is relatively short, and initially treatment discoveries were serendipitous. Early psoriasis therapies included arsenic and ammoniated mercury use in the 19th Century. In the first half of the 20th Century, anthralin and tar were discovered as effective psoriasis treatments. Corticosteroids were developed in the 1950s. These therapies were followed in the 1970s by use of methotrexate and PUVA on psoriasis. In the 1980s, psoriasis treatment discoveries included narrowband UVB, retinoids, and vitamin D therapies. From the 1990s to the present time, manipulating the immune system to treat psoriasis has been explored first with cyclosporine and more recently with targeted molecules.

19th Century – Arsenic and ammoniated mercury

Throughout history, arsenic has been utilized as both a poison and therapeutic. In 1806, Girdlestone reported on the efficacy of Fowler's Solution with 1% arsenic in treating many dermatologic conditions including psoriasis [1, 28]. With similar toxic potential, ammoniated mercury was used as a medication before the 20th Century [16, 29]. In 1876, Duhring recommended mercurial ointments to treat psoriasis [30].

1900–1950s – Anthralin and tar

In 1876, Squire inadvertently discovered anthralin as a treatment of psoriasis. Squire prescribed Goa powder, which was until then known only to be effective in ringworm, and the patient's psoriasis improved. The active ingredient of Goa powder is chrysarobin, also known as 2-methyl dithranol [31]. During World War I, this treatment was further refined, as a synthetic form of chrysarobin called antralin, or dithranol, was formed. In 1916, Unna reported the effectiveness of dithranol as an antipsoriatic treatment [32].

The next advancement in psoriasis treatment was coal tar. Hippocrates and other ancient physicians treated dermatologic conditions with pine tar and other types of tar. Coal tar became available when coal gas production developed in the late 19th Century, and Goeckerman found that coal tar was particularly useful in psoriasis therapy [33, 34]. Many observed that psoriasis improved with summer sun. In 1925, Goeckerman reported an additive benefit of coal tar and UVB radiation in psoriasis treatment [16, 35]. Goeckerman's method remained the mainstay of psoriasis treatment for decades. In 1953, Ingram reported the successful treatment of psoriasis with a combination of Unna and Goeckerman's modalities. He established the first day care center for psoriasis in which patients were treated with a tar bath, then UVB therapy, and lastly with 0.42% dithranol in Lassar's paste [36]. This treatment improved the morbidity of psoriasis for many patients, but was time intensive.

1950s – Corticosteroids

In the 1950s, the corticosteroid era began and revolutionized the treatment of many diseases. In 1950 Hench, Kendall, and Reichstein received the Nobel Prize for the development of cortisone [37, 38]. A mere 2 years later, Sulzberg and Witten reported that compound F, or hydrocortisone, was the first moderately successful topical corticosteroid in inflammatory skin diseases including psoriasis [39]. From that time forward, additional topical corticosteroid preparations were developed to treat inflammatory dermatoses such as psoriasis.

1970s – Methotrexate and PUVA

Although methotrexate was first developed in the 1950s, it was not used to treat psoriasis until the 1970s. In 1946, Farber developed aminopterin to treat leukemia [40]. Five years later, Gubner reported that aminopterin used in the treatment of rheumatoid arthritis also cleared psoriasis [23]. In 1958, Edmundsun and Guy introduced methotrexate, a more stable derivative of aminopterin with lower toxicity [41]. Investigators initially believed that folic acid antagonists prevented keratinocyte hyperproliferation, but later the effect on lymphocytes in psoriatic lesions was elucidated. In 1972, the FDA finally approved the use of methotrexate for psoriasis [42].

Also in the 1970s, PUVA therapy was reported to be effective in psoriasis. PUVA, based on the interaction between UV radiation and a photo-sensitizing chemical, has its own rich history [43]. The concept originated in about 1'500 BC when Egyptian healers treated vitiligo with a combination of sunlight and ingestion of plants known as psoralens, including fig and limes [44]. An article published in 1974 reported the efficacy of oral PUVA therapy in a group of patients with psoriasis [43]. Three years later, a multi-center study confirmed that most patients with psoriasis experienced clearing of their skin using oral PUVA [45]. Shortly after the development of oral PUVA, alternative bathwater delivery systems of psoralens were also created to minimize adverse effects associated with oral PUVA [46].

1980s – Narrowband UVB, retinoids, vitamin D

Although often therapeutically successful, PUVA therapy carries an increased risk of skin cancer. Therefore, further study of UVB therapy was undertaken. In 1981, Parrish and Jaenicke demonstrated that UVB wavelengths between 300 and 313 nm caused the greatest remission of skin lesions [47]. Subsequent trials reported that the 311 nm spectrum showed improved clearance of lesions with less erythema [48, 49].

In the 1980s, researchers also established the use of retinoids in psoriasis treatment. Prior to its use in psoriasis, in the 1960s physicians prescribed retinoids for hyperkeratosis and acne. At this time, first-generation and synthetic topical retinoids did not have significant antipsoriatic activity [50, 51]. In the early 1980s, reports demonstrated the efficacy of the second-generation retinoids etretinate and its derivative acitretin, in the treatment of psoriasis [52, 53]. Although etretinate is no longer available in the US due to its lipophilia and protracted adverse effects, acitretin has a shorter half life and remains an important therapy in psoriasis [54]. Third-generation acetylenic retinoids developed in the 1980s allowed for the production of a topical retinoid, tazarotene, with demonstrated anti-psoriatic efficacy [55].

The next class of drugs developed for psoriasis, vitamin D and its analogs, was also developed by chance observations in the 1980s. In 1985, a patient who received oral vitamin D3 for osteoporosis experienced dramatic improvement of his psoriasis [56]. The active form of vitamin D3 plays a part in the control of intestinal calcium absorption, bone mineralization, keratinocyte differentiation, keratinocyte proliferation, and immune modulation [57, 58]. Despite extensive research, the exact mechanism of action of vitamin D analogs remains unknown. In 1988, a topical form of vitamin D proved useful in the treatment of psoriasis [59].

1990s – Cyclic immunosuppressive medications

In 1997, cyclosporine was FDA approved for psoriasis treatment. Cyclosporine was isolated in 1969 from a fungus and was screened for antibiotic properties. In 1976, Borel reported immunosuppressive properties of cyclosporine in animal models [60]. Three years later, Cyclosporine A was used experimentally in transplant patients to prevent graft rejection, and psoriatic patients in these trials experienced relief of their lesions [24]. FDA approval was delayed until the 1990s due to concerns about toxicity. Cyclosporine is prescribed for severe psoriasis that is not responsive to other therapies [61].

Psoriasis treatment discoveries of today and tomorrow

Although our understanding of the immunological basis of psoriasis had expanded greatly by the turn of the Millennium, many details still remain unknown. Understanding of the role of immunology in psoriasis, together with the knowledge of protein engineering techniques, has given us the capability to manufacture specific proteins that can selectively alter the immunological processes in psoriasis. These therapies continue to improve the treatment of psoriasis and shed further light into its pathogenesis.

Beginning in January of 2003, a number of biologic agents were approved by the FDA for the treatment of psoriasis including alefacept, efalizumab, etanercept and infliximab. Alefacept binds to CD2 to prevent the activation of T lymphocytes in psoriasis [27, 62], while efalizumab, binds to CD11 to inhibit T cell activation and migration into the skin [63]. Both of these therapies strengthened the understanding of the role of T lymphocytes in psoriasis. Tumor necrosis factor inhibitors also demonstrated efficacy in the treatment of psoriasis [64]. The efficacy and mechanism of etanercept, infliximab and adalimumab suggest that psoriasis pathophysiology also involves immunologic mediators in addition to T cells. Discovery of these biologic therapies opens the door of our understanding of psoriasis. The quest for developing additional biologics for the treatment of psoriasis and other immune-mediated diseases continues, and it will be the role of clinicians to measure the potential advantages of each therapy for individual patients [65].

Our understanding of psoriasis and ability to treat this disease has evolved tremendously in the past few decades. We not only recognize psoriasis as distinct from leprosy and other inflammatory disorders, but are beginning to more fully understand its pathophysiology. More importantly, our ability to treat patients and improve their quality of life has progressed. Although we initially stumbled upon treatments by chance, we are now developing targeted therapies. These innovative therapeutics not only improve patient symptoms, but also help elucidate the pathophysiology of psoriasis and other immune-mediated diseases. The rich history of our understanding of psoriasis and its treatment serves as inspiration for continued discovery about psoriasis and its therapy.

References

1 Bechet PE (1936) Psoriasis, a brief historical review. *Arch Dermatol Syph* 33: 327–334
2 Hebra F (1868) *On disease of the skin.* New Sydenham Society, London
3 Fox H (1915) Dermatology of the ancients. *JAMA* 65: 469
4 Sutton RL (1986) *Sixteenth century physician and his methods mercurialis on diseases of the skin.* The Lowell Press, Kansas City, MO
5 Pusey WA (1933) *The history of dermatology.* Charles C Thomas, Springfield, IL
6 Glickman FS (1986) Lepra, psora, psoriasis. *J Am Acad Dermatol* 14(5 Pt 1): 863–866
7 Celsus AC (1837) *De re medica.* East Portwine, London
8 Willan, R (1809) *On Cutaneous Diseases.* Kimber and Conrad, Philadelphia

9 Rayer P (1835) *Treatises on diseases of the skin.* 2nd ed. J.B. Bailliere, London
10 Gibert CM (1840) *Traite pratique des maladies speciales de la peau.* 2nd ed. Germer-Bailliere, Paris
11 Wilson E (1863) *Diseases of the skin.* Blanchchard and Lea, Philadelphia
12 Fox T (1871) *Skin diseases: Their description, pathology, diagnosis, and treatment.* William Wood and Co, New York
13 Milton JL (1872) *Diseases of the skin.* Robert Hardwicke, London
14 Crissey JT, Parish LC, Shelley WB (1981) *The dermatology and syphilology of the nineteenth century.* Praiger Publishers, New York
15 Hebra on F, Kaposi M (1876) *Lehrbuch der Hautkrankheiten.* Ferdinanand Euke, Stuttgart
16 Fry L (1988) Psoriasis. *Br J Dermatol* 119(4): 445–461
17 Farber EM (1982) Historical Commentary. In: EM Farber, AJ Cox, L Nall, PH Jacobs (eds): *Psoriasis: proceedings of the Third International Symposium, Stanford University, 1981.* Third ed. Grune and Stratton, New York, 7–11
18 Köbner H (1876) Zur Aetiologie der Psoriasis. *Vjschr Dermatol* 3: 559–561
19 von Zumbusch LR (1910) Psoriasis und pustuloses exanthem. *Archives of Dermatology and Syphiliology* 99: 335–346
20 Woronoff DL (1926) Die peripheren Veränderungen der Haut um die Effloreszenzen der Psoriasis vulgaris und Syphilis corymbosa. *Dermatologische Wochenschrift* 82: 249–257
21 VanScott EJ, Ekel TM (1963) Kinetics of hyperplasia in psoriasis. *Arch Dermatol* 88: 373–381
22 Weinstein GD, Van Scott EJ (1966) Turnover time of human normal and psoriatic epidermis by autoradiographic analysis. *J Inves Dermatol* 45: 561–567
23 Gubner R (1951) Effect of aminopterin on epithelial tissues. *AMA Arch Derm Syphilol* 64(6): 688–699
24 Mueller W, Herrmann B (1979) Cyclosporin A for psoriasis. *N Engl J Med* 301(10): 555
25 Bjerke JR, Krogh HK, Matre R (1978) Characterization of mononuclear cell infiltrates in psoriatic lesions. *J Invest Dermatol* 71(5): 340–343
26 Baker BS, Swain AF, Fry L, Valdimarsson H (1984) Epidermal T lymphocytes and HLA-DR expression in psoriasis. *Br J Dermatol* 110(5): 555–564
27 Schon MP, Boehncke WH (2005) Psoriasis. *N Engl J Med* 352(18): 1899–1912
28 Girdlestone T (1806) Observations on the effects of Dr. Fowler's mineral solution in lepra and other diseases. *Med Phys J London* 15: 298–301
29 Farber EM (1992) History of the treatment of psoriasis. *J Am Acad Dermatol* 27(4): 640–645
30 Duhring LA (1876) *Atlas of skin diseases.* JB Lippincot and Co, Philadelphia
31 Squire B (1876) Treatment of psoriasis by an ointment of chrysophanic acid. *BMJ* 819–920
32 Unna PG (1916) Cignolin als Heilmittel der Psoriasis. *Dermatologische Wochenschrift* 6: 116–137, 151–163, 175–183
33 Hjorth N, Norgaard M (1991) Tars. In: HH Roenigk, HL Maibach (eds): *Psoriasis.* Marcel Dekker, New York, 473–479
34 Squire B (1878) *Atlas of skin diseases.* JandA Churchill, London
35 Goeckerman WH (1925) The treatment of psoriasis. *Northwest Med* 25: 229–231
36 Ingram JT (1953) The approach to psoriasis. *BMJ* 2: 591–593
37 Lundberg IE, Grundtman C, Larsson E, Klareskog L (2004) Corticosteroids – from an idea to clinical use. *Best Pract Res Clin Rheumatol* 18(1): 7–19
38 Hench PS, Kendall EC, Slocumb CH, Polley HF (1950) Effects of cortisone acetate and pituitary ACTH on rheumatoid arthritis, rheumatic fever and certain other conditions. *Arch Med Interna* 85(4): 545–666
39 Sulzberger MB, Witten VH (1952) The effect of topially applied compound F in selected dermatoses. *J Invest Dermatol* 19: 101–102
40 Farber S, Diamond L, Mercer R, Sylvester R, Wolff V (1946) Temporary remissions in acute leukemia in children produced by folic acid antagonist 4-amethopteroylglutamic acid (aminopterin). *N Engl J Med* 238: 787–793
41 Edmundson WF, Guy WB (1958) Treatment of psoriasis with folic acid antagonists. *AMA Arch Derm* 78(2): 200–203
42 Roenigk HH Jr, Maibach HI, Weinstein GD (1973) Use of methotrexate in psoriasis. *Arch Dermatol* 105(3): 363–365
43 Parrish JA, Fitzpatrick TB, Tanenbaum L, Pathak MA (1974) Photochemotherapy of psoriasis with oral methoxsalen and longwave ultraviolet light. *N Engl J Med* 291(23): 1207–1211

44 Benedetto AV (1977) The psoralens: An historical perspective. *Cutis* 20: 469–471
45 Melski JW, Tanenbaum L, Parrish JA, Fitzpatrick TB, Bleich HL (1977) Oral methoxsalen photochemotherapy for the treatment of psoriasis: A cooperative clinical trial. *J Invest Dermatol* 68(6): 328–335
46 Fischer T, Alsins J (1976) Treatment of psoriasis with trioxsalen baths and dysprosium lamps. *Acta Derm Venereol* 383–390
47 Parrish JA, Jaenicke KF (1981) Action spectrum for phototherapy of psoriasis. *J Invest Dermatol* 76: 359–361
48 Green C, Ferguson J, Lakshmipathi T, Johnson BE (1988) 311 nm UVB phototherapy – an effective treatment for psoriasis. *Br J Dermatol* 119(6): 691–696
49 Picot E, Meunier L, Picot-Debeze MC, Peyron JL, Meynadier J (1992) Treatment of psoriasis with a 311-nm UVB lamp. *Br J Dermatol* 127(5): 509–512
50 Wolbach SB, Howe PR (1925) Tisse changes following deprivation of fat-solbe A-vitamin. *J Experimental Med* 42: 753–778
51 Stuttgen G (1962) Zur Lokalbehandlung von Keratosen mit Vitamin A-Säure. *Dermatologica* 124: 65–80
52 Tsambaos D, Orfanos CE (1981) Chemotherapy of psoriasis and other skin disorders with oral retinoids. *Pharmacol Ther* 14(3): 355–374
53 Ward A, Brogden RN, Heel RC, Speight TM, Avery GS (1984) Isotretinoin. A review of its pharmacological properties and therapeutic efficacy in acne and other skin disorders. *Drugs* 28(1): 6–37
54 Ellis CN, Voorhees JJ (1987) Etretinate therapy. *J Am Acad Dermatol* 16(2, Part 1): 267–291
55 Weinstein GD (1996) Safety, efficacy and duration of therapeutic effect of tazarotene used in the treatment of plaque psoriasis. *Br J Dermatol* 135 Suppl 49: 32–36
56 Morimoto S, Kumahara Y (1985) A patient with psoriasis cured by 1 alpha-hydroxyvitamin D3. *Med J Osaka Univ* 35(3–4): 51–54
57 Smith EL, Walworth NC, Holick MF (1986) Effect of 1 alpha,25-dihydroxyvitamin D3 on the morphologic and biochemical differentiation of cultured human epidermal keratinocytes grown in serum-free conditions. *J Invest Dermatol* 86(6): 709–714
58 Kragballe K, Wildfang IL (1990) Calcipotriol (MC 903), a novel vitamin D3 analogue stimulates terminal differentiation and inhibits proliferation of cultured human keratinocytes. *Arch Dermatol Res* 282(3): 164–167
59 Kragballe K, Beck HI, Sogaard H (1988) Improvement of psoriasis by a topical vitamin D3 analogue (MC 903) in a double-blind study. *Br J Dermatol* 119(2): 223–230
60 Borel JF, Feurer C, Gubler HU, Stahelin H (1976) Biological effects of cyclosporin A: A new antilymphocytic agent. *Agents Actions* 6(4): 468–475
61 Griffiths CE, Dubertret L, Ellis CN, Finlay AY, Finzi AF, Ho VC, Johnston A, Katsambas A, Lison AE, Naeyaert JM et al. (2004) Ciclosporin in psoriasis clinical practice: An international consensus statement. *Br J Dermatol* 150 Suppl 67: 11–23
62 Ellis CN, Krueger GG (2001) Alefacept Clinical Study Group. Treatment of chronic plaque psoriasis by selective targeting of memory effector T lymphocytes. *N Engl J Med* 345(4): 248–255
63 Kupper TS (2003) Immunologic targets in psoriasis. *N Engl J Med* 349(21): 1987–1990
64 Leonardi CL, Powers JL, Matheson RT, Goffe BS, Zitnik R, Wang A, Gottlieb AB, Etanercept Psoriasis Study Group (2003) Etanercept as monotherapy in patients with psoriasis. *N Engl J Med* 349(21): 2014–2022
65 Lebwohl MG (2005) Advances in psoriasis. *Arch Dermatol* 141(12): 1589–1590

The pathophysiology of psoriasis

Marissa D. Newman[1] and Jeffrey M. Weinberg[2]

[1] *UMDNJ-Robert Wood Johnson Medical School New Jersey, New Jersey, 08902, USA*
[2] *Department of Dermatology, St. Luke's-Roosevelt Hospital Center and Beth Israel Medical Center, New York, 10025, USA*

Introduction

The past 25 years of research and clinical practice have revolutionized our understanding of the pathogenesis of psoriasis as the dysregulation of immunity triggered by environmental and genetic stimuli. Psoriasis was originally regarded as a primary disorder of epidermal hyperproliferation. However, experimental models and clinical results from immunomodulating therapies have refined this perspective in conceptualizing psoriasis as a genetically programmed pathologic interaction between resident skin cells, infiltrating immunocytes and a host of proinflammatory cytokines, chemokines and growth factors produced by these immunocytes. Two populations of immunocytes and their respective signaling molecules collaborate in the pathogenesis: innate immunocytes, mediated by antigen presenting cells (including natural killer T lymphocytes, Langerhans cells and neutrophils) and acquired or adaptive immunocytes, mediated by mature CD4+ and CD8+ T lymphocytes in the skin. Such dysregulation of immunity and subsequent inflammation is responsible for the development and perpetuation of the clinical plaques and histological inflammatory infiltrate characteristic of psoriasis.

Although psoriasis is considered to be an immune mediated disease in which intralesional T lymphocytes and their proinflammatory signals trigger primed basal layer keratinocytes to rapidly proliferate, debate and research focus on the stimulus that incites this inflammatory process. While psoriasis may represent an autoimmune reaction, researchers have not isolated self-antigens or defined the specificity of the auto-reactive skin lymphocytes. Our current understanding considers psoriasis to be triggered by exogenous or endogenous environmental stimuli in genetically susceptible individuals. Such stimuli include Group A streptococcal pharyngitis, viremia, allergic drug reactions, antimalarial drugs, lithium, beta blockers, interferon alpha, withdrawal of systemic corticosteroids, local trauma (Köbner's phenomenon) and emotional stress, as these correlate with the onset or flares of psoriatic lesions. Psoriasis genetics centers on susceptibility loci and corresponding candidate genes, particularly the psoriasis susceptibility (PSORS) 1 locus on the major histocompatibility (MHC) class I region. Current research on the pathogenesis of psoriasis examines the complex interactions between immunologic mechanisms, environmental stimuli and genetic susceptibility. After discussing the clinical presentation and histopathologic features of psoriasis, we will review the pathophysiology of psoriasis through noteworthy developments including serendipitous observations, reactions to therapies, clinical trials and animal model systems that have shaped our view of the disease process.

Clinical presentations

There are multiple patterns of psoriasis including plague, guttate, pustular, inverse and erythrodermic. Approximately 80% of patients present with plaque psoriasis which is clinically characterized by well demarcated erythematous plaques with overlying scales. These lesions are distributed symmetrically and frequently occur on the elbows, knees, lower back and scalp. These plaques can be intensely pruritic and bleed when manipulated, referred to as the Auspitz sign.

In addition to the classic skin lesions, approximately 23% of psoriasis patients develop psoriatic arthritis with a 10 year latency after diagnosis of psoriasis [1]. The distal interphalangeal (DIP), wrist, sacroiliac (SI) and knee joints are most commonly affected with swelling, stiffness and loss of function. With longstanding disease, bone changes can be demonstrated on radiographs and bone scans. Psoriatic arthritis patients are rheumatoid factor negative which differentiates them from patients with rheumatoid arthritis. Additionally, nail involvement occurs in 30–50% of patients and may clinically resemble a fungal infection, with pitting, onycholysis, thickening, with hyperkeratotic debris under the nail plate [1].

Histopathology

The histology of psoriatic plaques is distinguished by excessive epidermal growth termed psoriasiform hyperplasia. This pattern includes a markedly thickened skin or acanthosis, elongated downward extensions of the epidermis into the dermis or rete pegs and aberrant keratinocyte differentiation. Mitotic figures are visible at the basal layer of keratinocytes demonstrating rapid proliferation and maturation responsible for incomplete terminal differentiation. Thus, keratinocytes retain their nuclei as visualized in the parakeratotic stratum corneum. The granular layer of the epidermis is also depleted. Additionally, the rapidly proliferating keratinocytes fail to secrete lipids that normally adhere the corneocytes to each other, thereby producing the classic scale of a psoriatic plaque. The tortuous and dilated dermal blood vessels are responsible for the erythema exhibited by psoriatic plaques.

In addition to epidermal hyperproliferation, an inflammatory infiltrate distinguishes psoriatic skin. Collections of neutrophils termed Munro's abscesses are found within the stratum corneum. Furthermore, an influx of T cells is found in both the epidermis and dermis along with increased numbers of dermal dendritic cells, macrophages and mast cells. These unique histologic features of the psoriatic plaque represent the starting line for researchers determining the mechanisms that underlie the pathophysiology of psoriasis.

Principles of immunity

The immune system, intended to protect its host from foreign invaders and unregulated cell growth, employs two main effector pathways. These are the innate and acquired or adaptive immune responses, both of which contribute to the pathophysiology of psoriasis [2]. Innate immunity responses occur within minutes to hours, but fail to develop memory for when the antigen is encountered again. However, adaptive immunity responses take days to weeks to respond after challenged with an antigen. The adaptive immune cells have the capacity to respond to a greater range of antigens and develop immunologic memory via rearrangement of antigen receptors on B and T cells. These specialized B and T cells can subsequently be promptly mobilized and differentiated into mature effector cells that protect the host from a foreign pathogen. Innate and adaptive immune responses are highly intertwined; they can initiate, perpetuate and terminate the immune mechanisms responsible for inflammation. They can modify the nature of the immune response by altering the relative proportion of type 1 helper T (T_H1) cells *versus* type 2 helper (T_H2) cells and their respective signaling molecules. A T_H1 response is essential for a cellular immunologic reaction to an antigen or cellular immunity, while a T_H2 response promotes IgE synthesis, eosinophilia, mast cell maturation and humoral immunity. The innate and adaptive immune responses employ common effector molecules such as chemokines and cytokines that are essential in mediating an immune response.

Implicating dysregulation of immunity

Our present appreciation of the pathogenesis of psoriasis is based on the history of trial and error therapies, serendipitous discoveries and the current immune targeting drugs used in a variety of chronic inflammatory conditions including rheumatoid arthritis, ankylosing spondylitis and inflammatory bowel disease. Before the mid 1980s research focused on the hyperproliferative epidermal cells as the primary pathology as a markedly thickened epidermis was indeed demonstrated on histological specimens. Altered cell cycle kinetics were thought to be the culprit behind the hyperkeratotic plaques. Thus, initial treatments centered on oncologic and antimitotic therapies used to arrest keratinocyte proliferation with agents such as arsenic, ammoniated mercury and methotrexate [3].

However, a paradigm shift from targeting epidermal keratinocytes to immunocyte populations occurred when a patient receiving cyclosporine to prevent transplant rejection noted clearing of psoriatic lesions in the 1980s [4]. Cyclosporine was observed to inhibit mRNA transcription of T cell cytokines thereby implicating immunologic dysregulation, specifically T cell hyperactivity, in the pathogenesis of psoriasis [5]. However, the concentrations of oral cyclosporine reached in the epidermis exerted direct effects on keratinocyte proliferation and lymphocyte function in such patients [6]. Thus it begged the question as to whether the keratinocytes or the lymphocytes drove the psoriatic plaques. The use of an interleukin (IL)-2 diptheria toxin-fusion protein, denileukin diftitox, specific for activated T cells with high affinity IL-2 receptors and nonreactive with keratinocytes distinguished which cell type was responsible. Used as a single agent, the targeted T cell toxin provided clinical and histological clearing of psoriatic plaques. Thus, T lymphocytes rather than keratinocytes were recognized as the definitive driver behind the psoriatic plaques [7].

Additional studies have demonstrated that treatments that induce prolonged clearing of psoriatic lesions without continuous therapy such as psoralens plus ultraviolet A irradiation (PUVA) decreased the numbers of T cells in plaques by at least 90% [8]. However, treatments that require continual therapy for satisfactory clinical results such as cyclosporine and etretinate, simply suppress T cell activity and proliferation [9, 10].

Further evidence has linked cellular immunity with the pathogenesis of psoriasis. Natural killer T (NKT) cells were shown to be involved through using severe combined immunodeficient (SCID) mouse model. NKT cells were injected into prepsoriatic skin grafted on immunodeficient mice creating a psoriatic plaque with an immune response showing cytokines from type 1 helper T cells (T_H1) rather than type 2 helper cells (T_H2) [11]. When psoriatic plaques were treated topically with the toll-like receptor (TLR) 7 agonist imiquimod, aggravation and spreading of the plaques were noted. The exacerbation of psoriasis was accompanied by an induction of lesional T_H1 type interferon produced by plasmacytoid dendritic cell (DC) precursors. Plasmacytoid DCs were observed to compose up to 16% of the total dermal infiltrate in psoriatic skin lesions based on their coexpression of BDCA2 and CD123 [12]. Additionally, cancer patients being treated with interferon (IFN)-alpha experienced induction of psoriasis [13]. Moreover, patients being treated for warts with intralesional IFN-alpha developed psoriatic plaques in neighboring prior asymptomatic skin [14]. Patients with psoriasis treated with IFN-gamma, a T_H1 cytokine type, also experienced the development of new plaques correlating with the sites of injection [15]. Thus, while epidermal hyperproliferation is the major phenotypic abnormality of psoriatic skin, these studies and growing evidence have shifted our focus of research to the immunologic and inflammatory mechanisms that promote this ultimate cutaneous manifestation of psoriasis.

Intralesional T lymphocytes

Psoriatic lesions contain a host of innate immunocytes such as antigen presenting cells (APCs), natural killer (NK) cells and neutrophils as well as adaptive T cells and an inflammatory infiltrate. These cells include CD4 and CD8 subtypes in which the CD8+ cells predominate in the epidermis while CD4+ cells show preference for the dermis [16]. There are two groups of CD8+ cells: one group migrates to the epidermis expressing the integrin CD103 while the other group is found in the dermis, but may be headed to or from the epidermis. The CD8+ cells residing in the epidermis that express the integrin CD103 are capable of interacting with E-cadherin which enables these cells to travel to the epidermis and bind resident cells. Immunophenotyping reveals that these mature T cells represent chiefly activated memory cells including CD2+, CD3+, CD5+, CLA, CD28 and CD45RO+ [17]. Many of these cells express the activation markers such as HLA-DR, CD25 and CD27 in addition to the T cell receptor (TCR).

T lymphocyte stimulation

Both mature CD4+ and CD8+ T cells can respond to the peptides presented by APCs. While the specific antigen that these T cells are reacting to has not yet been elucidated, several antigenic stimuli have been proposed. These include self proteins, microbial pathogens and microbial superantigens. The premise that self reactive T lymphocytes may contribute to the disease process is derived from the molecular mimicry theory in which an exuberant immune response to a pathogen produces cross-reactivity with self antigens. Considering that infections have been associated with the onset of psoriasis, this theory merits consideration. However, it has also been observed that T cells can be activated without antigens or superantigens, but rather with direct contact with accessory cells [18]. No single theory has clearly emerged, and thus researchers continue to search for the inciting stimulus that triggers the T lymphocyte and whether T cells are reacting to a self or non-self derived antigen.

T lymphocyte signaling

T cell signaling is a highly coordinated process in which T lymphocytes, of the T_HI variety, recognize antigens via presentation by mature APCs in the skin rather than the lymphoid tissues. Such APCs expose antigenic peptides via MHC I or II molecules for which receptors are present on the T cell surface. The antigen recognition complex at the T cell and APC interface in concert with a host of antigen independent costimulatory signals described below regulate T cell signaling and are referred to as the immunologic synapse. The antigen presentation and network of costimulatory and adhesion molecules optimize T cell activation which subsequently supports the production of growth factors and cytokines. These growth factors sustain neoangiogenesis, stimulate epidermal hyperproliferation, alter epidermal differentiation and decrease susceptibility to apoptosis that characterize the erythematous hypertrophic scaling lesions of psoriasis [19]. Furthermore, the cytokines produced from the immunologic response, such as tumor necrosis factor (TNF)-alpha and interferon (IFN)-gamma and IL-2, are correspond to cytokines that are upregulated in psoriatic plaques [20].

Integral components of the immunologic synapse complex include costimulatory signals including CD28, CD40, CD80 and CD86, and adhesion molecules such as cytotoxic T lymphocyte antigen 4 and lymphocyte function associated antigen (LFA)-1 that possess corresponding receptors on the T cell. These molecules play a key role in T cell signaling as their disruption has been shown to decrease T cell responsiveness and associated inflammation. The B7 family of molecules routinely interacts with CD28 T cells in order to costimulate T cell activation. Cytotoxic T lymphocyte antigen 4 immunoglobulin, an antibody on the T cell surface, targets B7 and interferes with signaling between B7 and CD28. In psoriatic patients, this blockade was demonstrated to attenuate the T cell response and correlated with a clinical and histologic decrease in psoriasiform hyperplasia [21]. Biological therapies that disrupt the LFA-1 component of the immunologic synapse have also demonstrated efficacy in the treatment of psoriasis. Alefacept is a human LFA-3 fusion protein that binds CD2 on T cells and blocks the interaction between LFA-3 on APCs and CD2 on memory CD45RO+ T cells and induces apoptosis of such T cells. Efalizumab is a human monoclonal antibody to the CD11 chain of LFA-1 that blocks the interaction between LFA-1 on the T cell and intercellular adhesion molecule (ICAM)-1 on an APC or endothelial cell. Both alefacept and efalizumab have demonstrated significant clinical reduction of psoriatic lesions, and alefacept has been shown to produce disease remission for up to 18 months after discontinuation of therapy [22–24]. Alefacept and efalizumab have been approved in the US and the EU for the treatment of moderate to severe psoriasis.

Natural killer T cells

Natural killer (NK) T cells represent a subset of CD3+ T cells present in psoriatic plaques. While NKT cells possess a TCR, they differ from T cells by displaying NK receptors comprised of lectin and immunoglobulin families. These cells exhibit remarkable specificity and are activated upon recognition of glycolipids presented by CD1d molecules. This process occurs in contrast to CD4+ and CD8+ T cells, which due to their TCR diversity, respond to peptides processed by APCs and displayed on MHC molecules. NKT cells can be classified into two subsets: one group that expresses CD4 and preferentially produces T_H1 *versus* T_H2 type cytokines and another group that lacks CD4 and CD8 that only produces T_H1 type cytokines. The innate immune system employs NKT cells early in the immune response because of their direct cytotoxicity and rapid production of cytokines such as IFN-gamma and IL-4. IFN-gamma promotes a T_H1 inflammatory response, while IL-4 promotes the development T_H2 cells. Excessive or dysfunctional NKT cells have been associated with autoimmune diseases such as multiple sclerosis and inflammatory bowel disease as well as allergic contact dermatitis [25–27].

In psoriasis, NKT cells are located in the epidermis, closely situated to epidermal keratinocytes which suggests a role for direct antigen presentation. Furthermore, CD1d is overexpressed throughout the epidermis of psoriatic plaques whereas CD1d expression is confined to terminally differentiated keratinocytes. An *in vitro* study examining cytokine based inflammation demonstrative of psoriasis treated cultured CD1d-positive keratinocytes with IFN-gamma in the presence of alpha-galactosylceramide of the lectin family [28]. IFN-gamma was observed to enhance keratinocyte CD1d expression, and subsequently CD1d-positive keratinocytes were found to activate NK-T cells to produce high levels IFN-gamma while levels of IL-4 remained undetectable. The preferential production of IFN-gamma supports a T_H1 mediated mechanism regulated by NKT cells in the immunopathogenesis of psoriasis.

Dendritic cells

Dendritic cells are professional APCs that process antigens in the tissues in which they reside after which they migrate to local lymph nodes where they present their native antigens to T cells. This process allows the T cell response to be tailored to the appropriate antigens in the corresponding tissues. Immature dendritic cells that capture antigens mature via migrating to the T cell center of the lymph node where they present their antigens to either MHC molecules or the CD1 family. This presentation results in T cell proliferation and differentiation that correlates with the required type of T cell response. Multiple subsets of APCs including myeloid and plasmacytoid DCs are highly represented in the epidermis and dermis of psoriatic plaques as compared with normal skin [29]. When faced with specific viruses and bacteria, precursors to plasmacytoid DCs have been shown to produce high levels of T_H1 type cytokines such as IFN-alpha and -beta that are characteristic of psoriatic inflammation.

While DCs play a pivotal role in eliciting an immune response against a foreign invader, they also contribute to the establishment of tolerance. Throughout their maturation, DCs are continuously sensing their environment which shapes their production of T_H1 *versus* T_H2 type cytokines and subsequently the nature of the T cell response. When challenged with a virus, bacteria or unchecked cell growth, DCs mature into APCs. However, in the absence of a strong stimulus, DCs fail to mature into APCs, but rather present self peptides with MHC molecules thereby creating regulatory T cells involved in peripheral tolerance [30]. If this balance between immunogenic APCs and housekeeping T cells is upset, inflammatory conditions such as psoriasis can result.

Cytokines

Cytokines are low molecular weight glycoproteins that function as signals to produce inflammation, defense, tissue repair and remodeling, fibrosis, angiogenesis and restriction of neoplastic growth [31]. Cytokines are produced by immunocytes such as lymphocytes and macrophages as well as non-immunocytes such as endothelial cells and keratinocytes. Proinflammatory cytokines include IL-1, IL-2, IFN-gamma and TNF-alpha while anti-inflammatory cytokines include IL-4 and IL-10. A relative preponderance of T_H1 proinflammatory cytokines or an insufficiency of T_H2 anti-inflammatory cytokines induces local inflammation and recruitment of additional immunocyte populations which produce added cytokines [32]. A vicious cycle of inflammation occurs that results in cutaneous manifestations such as a plaque. Psoriatic lesions are characterized by a relative increase of T_H1 (IL-2, IFN-gamma TNF-alpha and TNF-beta) to T_H2 (IL-4, IL-5, IL-6, IL-9, IL-10 and IL-13) type cytokines. As discussed previously, NKT cells stimulated by CD1d over-expressing keratinocytes increase production of proinflammatory IFN-gamma without effect on the anti-inflammatory IL-4. In addition to the cytokines produced by T cells, APCs produce IL-18, IL-23 and TNF-alpha found in the inflammatory infiltrate of psoriatic plagues. Both IL-18 and IL-23 stimulate T_H1 cells to produce IFN-gamma. Clearly, a T_H1 type pattern governs the immune effector cells and their respective cytokines present in psoriatic skin.

TNF-alpha

Although a network of cytokines is responsible for the inflammation of psoriasis, TNF-alpha has been implicated as a master proinflammatory cytokine of the innate immune response due to its widespread targets and sources. TNF-alpha is produced by activated T cells, keratinocytes, NK cells, macrophages, monocytes, Langerhan's APCs and endothelial cells. TNF-alpha was originally observed to induce septic shock and tumor cell necrosis at higher concentrations as well as function as an immune mediator of local tissue insults at lower concentrations. Psoriatic lesions demonstrate high concentrations of TNF-alpha, while the synovial fluid of psoriatic arthritis patients demonstrates elevated concentrations of TNF-alpha, IL-1, IL-6 and IL-8 [33]. In psoriasis, TNF-alpha supports the expression of adhesion molecules (intercellular adhesion molecule (ICAM)-1 and P-and E-selectin), angiogenesis via vascular endothelial growth factor (VEGF), the synthesis of proinflammatory molecules (IL-1, IL-6, IL-8 and nuclear factor (NF)-kappaB) and keratinocyte hyperproliferation via vasoactive intestinal peptide (VIP) [34].

A role for TNF-alpha in psoriasis treatment was serendipitously discovered in a trial for Crohn's disease in which infliximab, a mouse human IgG1 anti-TNF-alpha monoclonal antibody, was observed to clear psoriatic plaques in a patient with both Crohn's disease and psoriasis [35]. Immunotherapies that target TNF-alpha, including infliximab, etanercept, and adalimumab, show significant efficacy in the treatment of psoriasis [36–38]. TNF-alpha is regarded as the driver the inflammatory cycle of psoriasis due to its numerous modes of production, capability to amplify other proinflammatory signals and efficacy and rapidity with which it produces clinical improvements in psoriasis.

Genetic basis of psoriasis

Psoriasis is a disease of overactive immunity in genetically susceptible individuals. Because patients exhibit varying skin phenotypes, extracutaneous manifestations and disease courses, multiple genes resulting from linkage disequilibrium are believed to be involved in the pathogenesis of psoriasis. A decade of genome-wide linkage scans have established that PSORS1 is the strongest susceptibility locus demonstrable through family linkage studies; PSORS1 is responsible for up to 50% of the genetic component of psoriasis [39]. More recently, human leucocyte antigen (HLA)-Cw6 has received the most attention as a candidate gene of the PSORS1 susceptibility locus on the MCH I region on chromosome 6p21.3 [40]. This gene may function in antigen presentation via MHC I which aids in the activation of the overactive T cells characteristic of psoriatic inflammation.

Genomic scans have shown additional susceptibility loci for psoriasis on chromosomes 1q21, 3q21, 4q32–35, 16q12, 17q25. Two regions on chromosome 17q were recently localized via mapping which demonstrated a 6 Mb separation thereby indicating independent linkage factors. Genes SLC9A3R1 and NAT9 are present in the first region while RAPTOR in demonstrated in the second region [41]. SLC9A3R1 and NAT9 are players that regulate signal transduction, the immunologic synapse and T cell growth. RAPTOR is involved in T cell function and growth pathways. Using these genes as an example, we can predict that the alterations of regulatory genes, even those yet undetermined, can enhance T cell proliferation and inflammation manifested in psoriasis.

Conclusion

Psoriasis is a complex disease whereby multiple exogenous and endogenous stimuli incite already heightened innate immune responses in genetically predetermined individuals. The disease process is a result of a network of cell types including T cells, dendritic cells and keratinocytes that, with the production of cytokines, generate a chronic inflammatory state. Our understanding of these cellular interactions and cytokines originates from developments, some meticulously planned, others serendipitous, in the fields of immunology, cell and molecular biology and genetics. Such progress has fostered the creation of targeted immune therapy that has demonstrated significant efficacy in psoriasis treatment. Further study of underlying the pathophysiology of psoriasis may provide additional targets for therapy.

References

1 Gottlieb A (1998) Psoriasis. *Disease Management and Clinical Outcomes* 1: 195–202
2 Gaspari A (2005) Innate and adaptive immunity and the pathophysiology of psoriasis. *J Am Acad Dermatol* 54: S67–S80
3 Barker J (1991) The pathophysiology of psoriasis. *Lancet* 338: 227–230
4 Nickoloff B, Nestle F (2004) Recent insights into the immunopathogenesis of psoriasis provide new therapeutic opportunities. *Sci Med* 113: 1664–1675
5 Bos J, Meinardi M, van Joost T, Huele F, Powles A, Fry L (1989) Use of cyclosporine in psoriasis. *Lancet* 23: 1500–1505
6 Khandke L, Krane J, Ashinoff R, Staiano-Coico L, Granelli-Piperno A, Luster A, Carter D, Krueger J, Gottlieb A (1991) Cyclosporine in psoriasis treatment: Inhibition of keratinocyte cell-cycle progression in G1 independent effects on transforming growth factor-alpha/epidermal growth factor receptor pathways. *Arch Dermatol* 127: 1172–1179
7 Gottlieb S, Gilleaudeau P, Johnson R, Estes L, Woodworth T, Gottlieb A, Krueger J (1995) Response of psoriasis to a lymphocyte-selective toxin (DAB389IL-2) suggests a primary immune, but not keratinocyte, pathogenic basis. *Nature Med* 1: 442–447
8 Vallat V, Gilleaudeau P, Battat L, Wolfe J, Nabeya R, Heftler N, Hodak E, Gottlieb A, Krueger J (1994) PUVA bath therapy strongly suppresses immunological and epidermal activation in psoriasis: a possible cellular basis for remittive therapy. *J Exp Med* 180: 283–296
9 Gottlieb A, Grossman R, Khandke L, Carter DM, Sehgal P, Fu S, Granelli-Piperno A, Rivas M, Barazani L, Krueger J (1992) Studies of the effect of cyclosporine in psoriasis *in vivo*: Combined effects on activated T lymphocytes and epidermal regenerative maturation. *J Invest Dermatol* 98: 302–309
10 Gottlieb S, Hayes E, Gilleaudeau P, Cardinale I, Gottlieb A, Krueger J (1996) Cellular actions of etretinate in psoriasis: Enhanced epidermal differentiation and reduced cell-mediated inflammation are unexpected outcomes. *J Cutaneous Pathol* 23: 404–418
11 Nickoloff B, Bonish B, Huang B, Porcelli S (2000) Characterization of a T cell line bearing natural killer receptors and capable of creating psoriasis in a SCID mouse model system. *J Dermatol Sci* 24: 212–225
12 Gillet M, Conrad C, Geiges M, Cozzio A, Thurlimann W, Burg G (2004) Psoriasis triggered by toll-like receptor 7 agonist imiquimod in the presence of dermal plasmacytoid dendritic cell precursors. *Arch Dermatol* 140: 1490–1495
13 Funk J, Langeland T, Schrumpf E, Hansen L (1991) Psoriasis induced by interferon-alpha. *Br J Dermatol* 125: 463–465
14 Shiohara T, Kobayahsi M, Abe K, Nagashima M (1988) Psoriasis occurring predominantly on warts: possible involvement of interferon alpha. *Arch Dermatol* 124: 1816–1821
15 Fierlbeck G, Rassner G, Muller C (1990) Psoriasis induced at the injection site of recombinant interferon gamma: results of immunohistologic investigations. *Arch Dermatol* 126: 351–355
16 Prinz J (2003) The role of T cells in psoriasis. *J Eur Acad Dermatol Venereol* 17 (Suppl): 1–5
17 Bos J, de Rie M (1999) The pathogenesis of psoriasis: immunological facts and speculations. *Immunology Today* 20: 40–46
18 Geginat J, Campagnaro S, Sallusto F, Lanzavecchia A (2002) TCR-independent proliferation and differentiation of human CD4+ T cell subsets induced by cytokines. *Adv Exp Med Bio* 512: 107–112
19 Kastelan M, Massari L, Brajac I (2006) Apoptosis mediated by cytolytic molecules might be responsible for maintenance of psoriatic plaques. *Med Hypotheses* 67: 336–337
20 Austin L, Ozawa M, Kikuchi T, Walters I, Krueger J (1999) The majority of epidermal T cells in Psoriasis vulgaris lesions can produce type 1 cytokines, interferon-gamma, interleukin-2, and tumor necrosis factor-alpha, defining TC1 (cytotoxic T lymphocyte) and TH1 effector populations: a type 1 differentiation bias is also measured in circulating blood T cells in psoriatic

patients. *J Invest Dermatol* 113: 752–759
21 Abrams J, Kelley S, Hayes E, Kikuchi T, Brown M, Kang S, Lebwohl M, Guzzo C, Jegasothy B, Linsley P et al. (2000) Blockade of T lymphocyte costimulation with cytotoxic T lymphocyte-associated antigen 4-immunoglobulin (CTLA4Ig) reverses the cellular pathology of psoriatic plagues, including the activation of keratinocytes, dendritic cells and endothelial cells. *J Exp Med* 192: 681–694
22 Lebwohl M, Christophers E, Langley R, Ortonne J, Roberts J, Griffiths C (2003) An international, randomized, double-blind, placebo-controlled phase 3 trial of intramuscular alefacept in patients with chronic plaque psoriasis. *Arch Dermatol* 139: 719–727
23 Krueger G, Ellis C (2003) Alefacept therapy produces remission for patients with chronic plaque psoriasis. *Br J Dermatol* 148: 784–788
24 Gordon K, Leonardi C, Tyring S, Gottlieb A, Walicke P, Dummer W, Papp K (2002) Efalizumab (anti-CD11a) is safe and effective in the treatment of psoriasis: Pooled results of the 12-week first treatment period from 2 phase III trials. *J Invest Dermatol* 119: 242
25 Singh A, Wilson M, Hong S, Olivares-Villagomez D, Du C, Stanic A, Joyce S, Sriram S, Koezuka Y, Van Kaer L (2001) Natural killer T cell activation protects mice against experimental autoimmune encephalomyelitis. *J Exp Med* 194: 1801–1811
26 Saubermann L, Beck P, De Jong Y, Pitman R, Ryan M, Kim H, Exley M, Snapper S, Balk S, Hagen S et al. (2000) Activation of natural killer T cells by alpha-glactosylceramide in the presence of CD1d provides protection against colitis in mice. *Gastroenterology* 119: 119–128
27 Campos R, Szczepanik M, Itakura A, Akahira-Azuma M, Sidobre S, Kronenberg M, Askenase P (2003) Cutaneous immunization rapidly activates liver invariant Valpha 14 NKT cells stimulating B-1 B cells to initiate T cell recruitment for elicitation of contact sensitivity. *J Exp Med* 198: 1785–1796
28 Bonish B, Jullien D, Dutronc Y, Huang B, Modlin R, Spada F, Porcelli S, Nickoloff B (2000) Overexpression of CD1d by keratinocytes in psoriasis and CD1d-dependent IFN-gamma production by NK-T cells. *J Immunol* 165: 4076–4085
29 Deguchi M, Aiba S, Ohtani H, Nagura H, Tagami H (2002) Comparison of the distribution and numbers of antigen-presenting cells among T-lymphocyte-mediated dermatoses: CD1a+, factor XIIIa+, and CD68+ cells in eczematous dermatitis, psoriasis, lichen planus and graft-*versus*-host disease. *Arch Dermatol Res* 294: 297–302
30 Bos J, de Rie M, Teunissen M, Piskin G (2005) Psoriasis: dysregulation of innate immunity. *Br J Dermatol* 152: 1098–1107
31 Trefzer U, Hofmann M, Sterry W, Asadullah K (2003) Cytokine and anticytokine therapy in dermatology. *Expert Opin Biol Ther* 3: 733–743
32 Nickoloff B (1991) The cytokine network in psoriasis. *Arch Dermatol* 127: 871–884
33 Gaspari A (2006) Innate and adaptive immunity and the pathophysiology of psoriasis. *J Am Acad Dermatol* 54 (Suppl 2): S67–S80
34 Victor F, Gottlieb A (2002) TNF-alpha and apoptosis: implications for the pathogenesis and treatment of psoriasis. *J Drugs Dermatol* 3: 264–275
35 Oh C, Das K, Gottlieb A (2000) Treatment with anti-tumour necrosis factor alpha (TNF-alpha) monoclonal antibody dramatically decreases the clinical activity of psoriasis lesions. *J Am Acad Dermatol* 42: 829–830
36 Reich K, Nestle FO, Papp K, Ortonne J, Evans R, Guzzo C, Li S, Dooley L, Griffiths C; EXPRESS study investigators (2005) Infliximab induction and maintenance therapy for moderate-to-severe psoriasis: a phase III, multicentre, double-blind trial. *Lancet* 366: 1367–1374
37 Leonardi C, Powers J, Matheson R, Goffe B, Zitnick R, Wang A, Gottlieb A (2003) Etanercept as monotherapy in patients with psoriasis. *N Engl J Med* 349: 2014–2022
38 Saini R, Tutrone W, Weinberg J (2005) Advances in therapy for psoriasis: an overview of infliximab, etanercept, efalizumab, alefacept, adalimumab, tazarotene, and pimecrolimus. *Curr Pharm Des* 11: 273–280
39 Rahman P, Elder J (2005) Genetic epidemiology of psoriasis and psoriatic arthritis. *Ann Rheum Dis* 64 (Suppl II): ii37–ii39
40 Elder J (2006) PSORS1: Linking genetics and immunology. *J Invest Dermatol* 126: 1205–1206
41 Krueger J, Bowcock A (2005) Psoriasis pathophysiology: current concepts of pathogenesis. *Ann Rheum Dis* 64 (Supp ll):ii30–ii36

Treatment of Psoriasis
Edited by J.M. Weinberg

Psoriasis and psoriatic arthritis: a clinical review

Allison J. Brown and Neil J. Korman

Department of Dermatology, Murdough Family Center for Psoriasis, University Hospitals Case Medical Center, 11100 Euclid Ave, Cleveland, OH 44106, USA

Introduction

Psoriasis is a common, systemic, inflammatory disease with genetic features that affects the skin and/or the joints and may be associated with significant morbidity. Psoriasis has a major impact on a patients' quality of life, which may not correlate with disease severity as measured by the physician. In recent years, extensive research on psoriasis has demonstrated this disease to be an immunologically mediated disorder. The development of targeted immunotherapeutic agents to treat psoriasis and psoriatic arthritis has been a critical advance in the care of patients with these conditions. This chapter will focus on the clinical features of psoriasis and psoriatic arthritis, as well as potential triggers and systemic associations. The ability to identify psoriasis and knowledge of the disease associations and triggers will aid in the physician's capacity to most effectively treat patients with this disease.

Clinical features

Types

Several variants of psoriasis are well characterized [1]. These include chronic plaque psoriasis, which is the most common variant, erythrodermic psoriasis, pustular psoriasis, inverse psoriasis, and guttate psoriasis.

Chronic plaque psoriasis

More than 90% of patients with psoriasis have chronic plaque psoriasis, also known as psoriasis vulgaris [1]. These patients have sharply demarcated erythematous plaques with overlying silvery-whitish scale. The scale typically extends almost to the peripheral edge and when removed leaves a glossy erythematous base with pinpoint bleeding (known as the Auspitz sign). Plaques may vary in size from under 1 cm to over 10 cm in diameter. Although psoriasis can affect any area of the body, lesions tend to occur symmetrically in areas with high rates of epidermal proliferation and most commonly affect the scalp, nails, extensor surfaces of the limbs, elbows, knees, umbilical, genital and sacral region. The face is typically spared.

Guttate psoriasis

Guttate psoriasis accounts for about 2% of patients with psoriasis [2], and most commonly develops in children and young adults after a β-hemolytic streptococcal infection. Lesions are the size and shape of water drops, typically 2–5 mm in diameter. While guttate lesions are often the initial presentation of psoriasis in genetically susceptible individuals, they can also develop in patients with known chronic plaque psoriasis. Adults more commonly go on to develop chronic plaque type psoriasis after presenting with guttate psoriasis. In contrast, the prognosis of children with guttate psoriasis is excellent, with spontaneous remission occurring usually over the course of weeks to months. Pharyngeal carriage of the offending streptococcus makes recurrence more likely [3].

Erythrodermic psoriasis

Erythrodermic psoriasis can develop gradually from chronic plaque disease or acutely with little preceding psoriasis. Generalized erythema covering nearly the entire body surface area with varying degrees of scaling is seen. Erythrodermic psoriasis may also occur as a rebound phenomenon precipitated by the rapid discontinuation of several different effective therapies including cyclosporine, methotrexate, efalizumab and oral, intravenous, or topical corticosteroids. Altered thermoregulatory properties of erythrodermic skin may lead to chills and hypothermia, and fluid loss may lead to dehydration. Fever and malaise are common. Laboratory abnormalities are nonspecific and include leukocytosis, eosinophilia, anemia, and decreased levels of serum albumin resulting from the loss of barrier function [4].

Pustular psoriasis

This subtype accounts for approximately 3% of total psoriasis patients [2]. Pustular psoriasis occurs as both a generalized form (generalized pustular psoriasis or the Von Zumbusch variant) and a localized form.

The typical patient who develops generalized pustular psoriasis has a history of chronic plaque psoriasis. Erythema begins abruptly on the palms, in the flexures, and at the edge of chronic psoriatic plaques. This is followed by sudden onset and painful generalized erythema with overlying patches of sterile macroscopic pustules usually a few millimeters in diameter. The pustules then coalesce into 'lakes of pus'. Fever, arthralgias, malaise, and diarrhea parallel skin symptoms. Reactive leukocytosis and electrolyte abnormalities, particularly hypocalcemia, are common. Recurrence of generalized pustular psoriasis is frequent. While the etiology is unknown, triggers include pregnancy (known as impetigo herpetiformis), abrupt discontinuation of corticosteroids, drugs, and infections.

Localized pustular psoriasis can be divided into two types: palmoplantar pustulosis and acrodermatitis continua of Hallopeau. Palmoplantar pustulosis presents as tender pustules on the palms and soles, often with painful fissuring. Similar to generalized pustular psoriasis, infections and drugs can also trigger the localized form. Acrodermatitis continua of Hallopeau usually starts on one finger or toe after an injury from minor trauma or infection. The skin over the area then becomes scaly and pustules develop. The nail may become involved and may eventually become dystrophic.

Inverse psoriasis

Inverse psoriasis is characterized by lesions in the intertriginous regions of skin folds. Because of the moist nature of these areas, the lesions tend to be sharply demarcated erythematous plaques without the characteristic scale. Common locations include the axillary, genital, perineal, intergluteal, and submammary areas. Flexural surfaces such as the antecubital fossae can exhibit similar lesions.

Nail psoriasis

Nail psoriasis can occur in all psoriasis subtypes. Fingernails are involved in approximately half of all psoriatic patients and toenails are involved in 35% [5]. The most common abnormality of the plate is 'pitting', or a few to multiple pencil point indentations on the dorsal nail plate, reflecting foci of psoriasis in the form of parakeratosis of the nail matrix. Transverse depressions of the nail plate are also due to intermittent foci of psoriasis. Localized tan-brown color changes known as 'oil drop spots' occur when leukocytes are present beneath the nail plate. Severe psoriatic involvement of the nail matrix can result in thickened nails with subungual hyperkeratosis and onychodystrophy. If the entire nail matrix is involved, a white crumbly poorly adherent nail is seen. Splinter hemorrhages may be seen and are due to increased capillary fragility. Pustular psoriasis may result in subungual pustules of the nail bed or matrix, which rarely can result in loss of the entire nail plate [6–8].

Oral psoriasis

Oral psoriasis occurs in 2–10% of psoriasis patients [9, 10]. The asymptomatic nature of oral lesions leads to a decreased tendency of physicians to examine the oral mucosa of psoriatic patients. Because oral lesions in psoriasis are nonspecific and infrequently biopsied, confirmatory evidence that these lesions actually represent psoriasis is lacking. Oral lesions of psoriasis are nonspecific and consist of migratory annular erythematous papules with hydrated whitish, gray, or yellow scale, and most often affect the tongue. Fissured tongue, stomatitis areata migrans, and benign migratory glossitis are the most frequent oral findings and they are found twice as frequently in psoriatic patients compared to controls [10, 11].

Psoriasis and itch

Psoriasis is derived from the Greek word *psora*, or itch. As many as 84% of patients report itch during the course of the disease and for some patients this symptom can be extremely disruptive to their daily lives [12]. One population-based study of patients with psoriasis demonstrated that 23% ranked itching as the "worst thing about psoriasis", more than any other symptom or appearance related problem, including pain, limitations on physical activity, or restrictions on clothing options [13]. While 80% of patients experience pruritus limited to psoriatic plaques, 20% of patients experience pruritus in non-lesional skin as well [14]. Paroxysmal pruritus may worsen at night, with dry skin, or in hot climates.

Potential triggers

Trauma

Trauma can trigger the exacerbation of psoriatic lesions or the development of new lesions (this is known as Köbner's phenomenon). In retrospective studies, 30–50% of patients give a history of having experienced Köbner's phenomenon [15]. Köbner's original description in 1872 suggests that the phenomenon is more frequently seen when the disease is active in other areas. Trauma as a trigger is more commonly seen in patients who develop psoriasis at an early age and those who require multiple therapies to control their disease [16].

Infections

Infections have long been recognized as important triggers for psoriasis exacerbations. Up to half of children with psoriasis have an exacerbation of their disease within 2 weeks following an upper respiratory infection [17, 18]. Infection with streptococcus pyogenes has a well-known association with guttate disease. Up to 85% of patients with an episode of acute guttate psoriasis show evidence of preceding streptococcal disease in the form of positive anti-streptolysin-O titers [18]. 55% of these patients gave a history of an acute upper respiratory infection in the few weeks preceding the eruption. Streptococcal infections can elicit exacerbations of other types of psoriasis and psoriatic arthritis as well. One study of 111 patients isolated streptococcus pyogenes in 13% of patients with a guttate flare of chronic plaque psoriasis, in 14% of patients with chronic plaque psoriasis, and in 26% of patients with acute guttate psoriasis, while 7% of the patients in the control group had streptococcus pyogenes isolated [19]. While no placebo-controlled trials have been performed, some reports suggest a possible role for antibiotics or tonsillectomy in the treatment of guttate psoriasis [3, 20]. Another important potential triggering factor for psoriasis is infection with the human immunodeficiency virus (HIV). The prevalence of psoriasis in patients with HIV infection is nearly 5%, about twice that seen in the general population. The clinical manifestations of psoriasis in HIV-infected patients are similar to those in non-HIV-infected patients. However, lesions of more than one subset of psoriasis are often found in the same HIV patient [21]. For example, a patient with chronic plaque psoriasis may go on to develop guttate or pustular lesions. Psoriasis may occur at any time in the course of an HIV infection and exacerbations tend to be longer and more frequent than those in otherwise healthy psoriasis patients [22]. Psoriasis does not seem to be related to the CD4 count, and there is a report of psoriasis remission in the terminal stages of the acquired immunodeficiency syndrome [23]. Rapid onset of acute eruptive psoriasis or frequent exacerbations should raise the possibility of underlying HIV disease [24].

Stress

Psychological distress is a causative or maintaining factor in disease expression for many patients with psoriasis. In one study, over 60% of psoriasis patients believed that stress was the principal factor in the cause of their psoriasis [25]. Farber and colleagues surveyed over 5'000 patients with psoriasis and 40% reported that their psoriasis occurred at times of worry and 37% experienced worsening psoriasis with worry [5]. Stress-induced relapse rates of up to 90% have been reported in children [17]. Additionally, patients with higher levels of psychological stress in the form of worry take longer to clear when given the same therapy as those with low levels of worry [26]. This study demonstrated that ‘low level worriers’ achieved clearing of their skin with PUVA (psoralen plus ultraviolet-A) a median of 19 days earlier than ‘high level worriers’ undergoing the same treatment [26]. Other studies reveal that cognitive-behavioral therapy in conjunction with medical therapy can lead to a significantly greater reduction in the severity of psoriasis than medical therapy alone [27, 28]. These findings support the concept that psychological stress may have a significant association with psoriasis exacerbations in some patients.

Medications

Several medications may trigger or worsen psoriasis. The most commonly reported medications that may trigger psoriasis include lithium, beta-blockers, non-steroidal anti-inflammatory drugs, tetracyclines, and antimalarials [29]. Several other medications that may worsen psoriasis include angiotensin converting enzyme (ACE) inhibitors, terbinafine, clonidine, iodine, amiodarone, penicillin, digoxin, interferon-alpha, and interleukin-2. The abrupt discontinuation of systemic or superpotent topical corticosteroids are well known triggers for psoriasis worsening. While these observations suggest the possibility that certain medications may trigger psoriasis worsening, no controlled trials have proved an association.

Alcohol and smoking

Alcohol and smoking have been implicated as triggering factors for psoriasis exacerbations. It is well documented that the prevalence of psoriasis is increased among patients who abuse alcohol [30]. However, conflicting evidence exists as to whether increased alcohol intake in psoriasis patients is a factor in the pathogenesis or whether having a chronic disorder like psoriasis leads to greater intake of alcohol in an attempt to self-medicate. For example, a study of 144 Finnish patients with psoriasis demonstrated that alcohol consumption in the previous 12 months was linked to the onset of psoriasis. This study suggests that psoriasis may lead to sustained alcohol abuse and that this alcohol intake may perpetuate the disease [31]. In contrast, another study of 55 female patients showed no association between alcohol consumption and the onset of psoriasis [32]. Further support of increasing alcohol abuse as a post-diagnosis condition was seen in a case-control study of 60 Australian twins who were discordant for psoriasis. In this study, no difference in alcohol consumption between discordant twins, either monozygotic or dizygotic, was discovered [33].

Mortality related to alcohol use in psoriasis has also been evaluated. A population-based study of over 5'000 patients followed for 22 years demonstrated that psoriatic patients have a significantly increased mortality rate when compared to a control group, especially deaths related directly or indirectly to alcohol consumption [34]. However, this study did not account for previous hepatotoxic psoriasis therapies or other medical conditions, and used the most severe psoriasis patients (those who required hospital admission for their psoriasis), suggesting that the elevated mortality rates attributed to these patients may have been overstated. In summary, alcohol consumption is more prevalent in psoriasis patients, and it may also increase the severity of psoriasis. The association of alcohol with the pathogenesis and exacerbation of psoriasis is less clear. Prolonged alcohol abuse may lead to alcoholic liver disease, and in that way may decrease treatment responsiveness and options, which may prolong exacerbations.

Similarly, it is well documented that patients with psoriasis are more likely than those without psoriasis to smoke. In one large cross-sectional study from Utah, 37% of psoriatic patients acknowledged they were smokers *versus* 25% smokers in the general population [35]. Conflicting data exist on whether smoking plays a role in the onset of psoriasis. The Finnish study of 144 patients mentioned above found no significant association between smoking and the onset of psoriasis [31]. Another study of 55 women demonstrated an increased smoking rate of psoriasis patients compared to controls, which predated the diagnosis [32]. More recently, Naldi et al. examined 560 patients and showed that the risk for developing psoriasis was the greater in former smokers and current smokers than in those who had never smoked [36]. Additionally, increased rates of smoking have been related to increased psoriasis severity [37]. In a three-year study of 818 patients, those that smoked greater than 20 cigarettes per day were at a two-fold increased risk for more severe psoriasis than those who smoked less than 10 cigarettes per day [37]. Despite the increased prevalence of smoking in psoriasis patients, the role of smoking as a definitive factor in the pathogenesis or progression of psoriasis remains unclear.

Obesity
The correlation between obesity and psoriasis is an area of some controversy. For example, one case-control study of patients with new onset psoriasis established that these patients were more likely to be obese that their counterparts visiting a dermatology clinic for another condition. This association held true when confounding factors of age, education, marital status, smoking, and alcohol were accounted for [36]. These results suggest that obesity may be a predisposing risk factor for the development of psoriasis. Herron and colleagues performed a cross-sectional study of psoriasis patients and found that the prevalence of obesity was doubled in psoriatic patients when compared to the general population [35]. However, they also found that when patients with psoriasis were asked to recollect their weights at the time of their diagnosis using a diagram to assess body image perception, patients with psoriasis were equally likely to be obese as their non-psoriatic counterparts. Herron and colleagues therefore concluded that obesity is likely a consequence, rather than a trigger of, psoriasis [35].

Estrogen
Elevated estrogen levels may serve as a trigger for psoriasis in some patients. Reports of new onset psoriasis at puberty, psoriasis worsened by estrogen therapy, and psoriasis that may be cyclical and related to menses, all suggest an etiologic role for elevated estrogen levels [38]. However, there have also been reports of psoriasis occurring or being exacerbated at the onset of menopause, which supports the opposite interpretation. While some patients report a worsening of psoriasis during pregnancy, nearly twice as many report improvement of their psoriasis during pregnancy [39, 40]. These findings demonstrate that the potential role of estrogen as a triggering factor for psoriasis is not entirely clear.

Disease course

Psoriasis encompasses a spectrum of cutaneous manifestations that vary from patient to patient and even in the same patient over time. While the majority of patients have chronic plaque psoriasis throughout the typically lifelong course of their disease, some patients may develop guttate, pustular, inverse or erythrodermic variants. Psoriatic plaques usually develop slowly over time. During exacerbations, however, plaques tend to enlarge more rapidly with an active peripheral edge of increasingly intense erythema and scale along with increases in plaque thickness. New psoriatic papules may arise in areas of normal skin surrounding the established plaques and coalesce with these to form increasingly larger plaques. Resolution of a plaque typically begins at its center. The end result of plaque clearance may be post-inflammatory hypo- or hyper-pigmentation that gradually fades giving way to normal-appearing skin. Complete remission of psoriasis for several years followed by reoccurrence of disease can occur.

Traditionally, chronic plaque psoriasis has been considered a single entity; however, recent evidence demonstrates that patients with thin and thick plaque psoriasis have differing clinical features [41]. As the complex genetics of psoriasis are elucidated, it is expected that these clinical variants will prove to have a genetic basis.

Epidemiology

Several large population-based studies in the US show a prevalence of between 1.4% [42] and 2.6% [13], with equal distribution between men and women.

Worldwide prevalence rates of psoriasis range from 0.6–4.8%, with rates varying between different countries and races [43, 44]. Asian-Americans have a prevalence of between 0.4% [5] and 0.7% [13], and African-Americans have a prevalence of between 0.45% [45] and 1.3% [46]. American-Indians have prevalence of 0.2% or less [5]. The prevalence of psoriasis in East Africa is about 3%, whereas West African countries have a prevalence of about 0.5% [47]. These significant differences in the prevalence of psoriasis from various regions of the world relate to the genetics of this disease as numerous studies have demonstrated that psoriasis is a genetic disease [1].

Although new onset psoriasis has been reported in all age groups from newborns to age 108 years [48], the disease tends to have a bimodal distribution of onset with the major peak occurring at 20–30 years of age, and a later smaller peak occurring at 50–60 years of age. The mean age of onset of psoriasis varies from study to study, but nearly 75% of patients with psoriasis have an onset before age 40, and 12% of patients have the onset of psoriasis at age 50–60 years of age [49, 50]. Patients with an older age of onset of psoriasis are less likely to have a family history of psoriasis than patients with a younger age of onset of psoriasis [50]. Familial concentration of psoriasis indicates an important role for hereditary factors; however, a 67% concordance in monozygotic twins suggests that environmental factors may also be an important component of psoriasis [51].

The age of onset of psoriasis may also be predictive of greater disease severity. One study of 1'774 patients revealed that the onset of psoriasis before the age of 30 is predictive of more extensive cutaneous involvement, nail involvement, and a relapsing-recurring clinical course. In contrast, onset of psoriasis after the age of 30 was predictive of chronic, continuously evolving plaque psoriasis as well as palmoplantar pustular disease [50, 52].

Systemic associations

Psoriasis has been associated with severe systemic diseases. Patients with ulcerative colitis are 3.8 times more likely and patients with Crohn's disease are 1.6 times more likely to have psoriasis than patients without inflammatory bowel disease (IBD). This data supports a common genetic link for these conditions and HLA-B27 is more common in patients with IBD and patients with psoriasis, particularly patients with pustular forms [53]. More recent studies confirm this association, and implicate T-helper-1 (TH-1) lymphocytes and the cytokines that they produce as the potential link. Therapies targeting tumor necrosis factor (TNF) have been effective in patients with Crohn's disease [54].

Recent studies suggest that patients with psoriasis have an increased risk for cardiovascular disease [55]. Patients with psoriasis are more frequently overweight [35, 56], have an increased incidence of diabetes [57–60], an increased incidence of hypertension [57, 60], and have an atherogenic lipoprotein profile at the onset of psoriasis with significantly higher VLDL cholesterol levels and HDLc levels that are independent of known confounding factors including age, sex, BMI, smoking, blood pressure, physical activity and alcohol consumption [55]. Recent studies suggest that the risk of myocardial infarction is increased in psoriasis with the greatest relative risk (~three-fold) occurring in younger patients with the most severe disease [58]. Whether traditional established cardiovascular risk factors alone (including the Framingham variables of age, sex, smoking history, blood pressure, total serum cholesterol, HDL cholesterol and family history) or potentially unique psoriasis-related risk factors are responsible for the increased cardiovascular risk in patients with psoriasis is unknown.

It is not clear whether psoriasis has any effects on the liver. Liver biopsies obtained from psoriasis patients prior to methotrexate therapy reveal a greater incidence of non-alcoholic steatohepatitis (fatty liver) than in the general population. In addition, psoriasis patients treated with methotrexate have more liver toxicity than patients with rheumatoid arthritis who are treated with methotrexate at similar dosages [61]. This observation may be explained by genetic tendencies, increased alcohol intake, or an increased risk of obesity and its associated non-alcoholic steatohepatitis that occurs in patients with psoriasis.

The occurrence of allergic contact dermatitis, asthma, urticaria, and atopic dermatitis is 3 to 25 times less frequent in psoriatic patients than in the general population [52]. Some reports suggest an incidence of atopic dermatitis as much as 50 times less than the general population [62]. This observation may be at least partially explained by the predominantly TH-1 response found in psoriasis as compared to the predominantly T-helper-2 (TH-2) response found in atopic dermatitis.

Patients with psoriasis may be at increased risk for the development of lymphoma. One study of over 2'700 patients with psoriasis followed for nearly 4 years showed an almost three-fold increased relative risk of developing any type of lymphoma compared to a control group, after accounting for sex and age [63]. While medications with a known risk of lymphoma had only been used in 1.55% of patients in this study, they cannot be completely eliminated as a potential confounding factor. Additionally, the patients in this study were all over age 65, and it is not known whether these findings would hold true for a younger cohort. A more recent retrospective study of 150'000 patients with psoriasis also demonstrates an increased risk of lymphoma, but suggests that the relative risk for all lymphomas is lower at 1.34. In this study, cutaneous T-cell lymphoma had a relative risk of 10.75 in patients with severe psoriasis, and Hodgkin's lymphoma had a relative risk of 3.18 in patients with severe psoriasis [64].

Psoriatic arthritis

Clinical features

Psoriatic arthritis was first defined by Moll and Wright in 1973 as "an inflammatory arthritis associated with psoriasis that usually presented with a negative serological test for rheumatoid arthritis [65]." Five clinical patterns of psoriatic arthritis have been used for classification: distal arthritis, asymmetric oligoarthritis, symmetric polyarthritis, arthritis with axial disease, and arthritis mutilans (Tab. 1). This classification scheme is most relevant early in the course of the disease and the subtype of psoriatic arthritis may change as the disease progresses [66]. The most commonly affected joints are the spine and the distal inter-phalangeal (DIP) joints [67], each being affected in 40–50% of cases. Spinal arthritis most often occurs after several years of disease in other joints. Distal arthritis and arthritis mutilans are the most specific manifestations of psoriatic arthritis [67, 68].

Arthritis mutilans is a very severe manifestation of chronic psoriatic arthritis that has been reported to occur in up to 16% of patients [69, 70]. Fortunately, the incidence of arthritis mutilans has become lower in recent years. Arthritis mutilans results from osteolysis of the phalanges and metacarpals of the hand or metatarsals of the feet. If severe, arthritis mutilans can result in 'telescoping' of the involved finger or toe [69, 71].

Involvement of the DIP joint is commonly seen in patients with nail disease [71]. Psoriatic onycho-pachydermo-periostitis is a type of psoriatic arthritis

Table 1. Moll and Wright's clinical patterns

Distal arthritis predominantly involving the distal inter-plalangeal joints with nail damage (5%)
Asymmetric oligoarthritis, with less than five joints affected in an asymmetrical pattern, generally affecting the distal inter-phalangeal, proximal inter-phalangeal and metatarsal phalangeal joints. (70%)
Symmetric polyarthritis, which resembles rheumatoid arthritis but is negative for rheumatoid factor (15%)
Arthritis mutilans, with destructive mutilation of the joints (5%)
Arthritis with or without peripheral joint involvement, in which spondyloarthropathy (axial spine disease), which may include both sacroilitis and spondylitis, is the principal articular manifestation (5%)

that includes psoriatic onychodystrophy, soft-tissue thickening above the terminal phalanx, and radiologic involvement of the phalanx including a periosteal reaction and bone erosions. Psoriatic onycho-pachydermo-periostitis may be explained by the anatomic relationship between nail and the terminal phalanx, whereby inflammation spreads from the dermis below the nail to the proximal bone through the fibrous septa, which join the two [72].

Radiographic and laboratory findings

Radiologic changes may not be seen in early psoriatic arthritis. Later in the disease, radiographic findings may be indistinguishable from those seen in rheumatoid arthritis. The most striking feature is the coexistence of erosive changes and new bone formation in the distal joints. Other changes commonly seen include lysis of terminal phalanges, periostitis and new bone formation at the site of the enthesis, and gross destruction of isolated joints. Ankylosis of the DIP and proximal inter-phalangeal (PIP) joint may lead to what has been termed 'claw' or 'paddle' deformities of the hands [69]. Shortening of the digits with telescoping of two bones or 'pencil in cup' deformities can occur in patients with the most severe disease [66]. In psoriatic arthritis, the relationship between radiologic changes and clinical damage is not always clear. Some patients have clinical manifestations of destructive arthritis without supporting radiographic evidence, while other patients may demonstrate radiologic evidence of joint erosions without obvious clinical manifestations of destructive psoriatic arthritis [73]. In a prospective registry of 655 patients with psoriatic arthritis, 81% of the joints evaluated demonstrated radiological damage first while 19% of the joints revealed clinical evidence of destructive arthritis first [73].

Laboratory findings are nonspecific. Rheumatoid factor (RF) is seen in 2–10% of patients. Antinuclear antibodies (ANA) are present at low titers (<1:40) in approximately half of patients, and in clinically significant titers (>1:80) in 14% of patients [70]. Anti-double stranded DNA (anti DS-DNA) antibodies are seen in 3% of psoriatic arthritis patients in the absence of exposure to anti-TNF therapies [74]. Both RF and ANA antibodies also occur in patients with psoriatic skin lesions who do not have arthritic lesions. Anti-cyclic citrullinated peptide (anti-CCP) antibodies, which are considered highly specific for rheumatoid arthritis, are seen in 8–16% of psoriatic arthritis patients [75, 76]. Other laboratory abnormalities may include anemia, elevated erythrocyte sedimentation rate, elevated C-reactive protein, hyperuricemia, hypergammaglobulinemia, and leukocytosis [70].

Other manifestations

Psoriatic arthritis is classified with the spondyloarthropathies because of the presence of spondylitis in up to 40% of patients [66]. Extra-articular features common to the spondyloarthropathies can be seen in psoriatic arthritis, such as mucous membrane lesions, diarrhea, aortic root dilation, and an association with HLA-B27 [66]. Conjunctivitis, iritis, and urethritis may also occur [69]. Rare manifestations of psoriatic arthritis include pulmonary fibrosis involving the upper lobes of the lungs and amyloidosis [69]. In contrast to the spondyloarthropathies, patients with psoriatic arthritis often have asymmetrical involvement of the spine, peripheral arthritic symptoms, and a lower level of pain and movement limitation [77].

Disease course

Psoriatic arthritis is a lifelong, relapsing, remitting condition with an insidious onset. In approximately 85% of patients, arthritis appears after the onset of skin disease, but the remaining 15% may experience psoriatic arthritis before or concurrently with the onset of skin disease [78]. Patients usually develop psoriasis an average of 10 years before the onset of psoriatic arthritis.

Patients with psoriatic arthritis initially present with pain in a large joint, such as the knee, or may have involvement of one or two interphalangeal joints and/or dactylitis (inflammation of a finger or toe). The classic presentation of psoriatic arthritis includes oligoarticular arthritis involving a large joint as well as one or two interphalangeal joints [69]. Patients experience pain and stiffness in the affected joints. More than 30 minutes of morning stiffness typically relieved by physical activity occurs in about half of psoriatic arthritis patients. The absence of morning stiffness does not make the diagnosis of psoriatic arthritis less likely. Arthritic symptoms commonly wax and wane in parallel with skin lesions, but permanent joint disease progression, destruction, and debilitation can be seen, especially if untreated. One study of early onset psoriatic arthritis involving 129 patients demonstrated that within 2 years of onset, 47% of patients had one or more joint erosions [79]. When patients with psoriatic arthritis are followed in the untreated state for 10 years, 50% will develop five or more deformed joints [80]. Patients with psoriatic arthritis who present with polyarticular involvement are most likely to show both clinical and radiological progression.

Physical examination during active arthritis may show joint line tenderness, effusions, and stress pain. Patients with psoriatic arthritis generally have less tenderness than patients with other inflammatory arthritides [81]. Pitting edema of the hands or feet can also be seen in patients with psoriatic arthritis. The edema is most commonly asymmetrical and often precedes or is the presenting symptom of psoriatic arthritis [82].

Soft tissue inflammation such as enthesitis (inflammation at ligament and tendon insertions), most commonly of the Achilles tendon, the plantar fascia at its insertion into the calcaneus and the pelvic bones [83] can be seen. Enthesitis occurs most commonly in the setting of monoarticular arthritis in the tendons near the joint affected [69]. Flexor tenosynovitis of the hands or other sites can also occur. Dactylitis, characterized by diffuse swelling of a whole digit, occurs in about half of patients with psoriatic arthritis and is associated with increased risk of progressive joint damage. This is thought to be due to inflammation of the soft tissues, tendon sheaths, and the adjacent joints and is often referred to as the 'sausage finger or toe'.

Epidemiology

Estimates of the prevalence of psoriatic arthritis among patients with psoriasis vary from as low as 5% to up to 30% [61, 84, 85], and men and women are equally affected [67, 78, 86, 87]. In spite of the observation that psoriatic arthritis affects men and women at equal rates, women are more likely to progress to severe disease than men [66].

Nail disease is the only clinical feature that identifies patients with psoriasis who are likely to develop arthritis and has been used as a diagnostic predictor of psoriatic arthritis [69]. 80–90% of patients with psoriatic arthritis have nail lesions whereas 46% of patients with psoriasis who do not have psoriatic arthritis have nail changes [88, 89].

A family history of psoriatic arthritis, disease onset before age 20, the presence of certain HLA types, erosive or polyarticular disease, and extensive skin involvement have all been associated with a poor prognosis for patients with psoriatic arthritis [69, 78, 79].

Comparison of psoriatic arthritis to rheumatoid arthritis

Because rheumatoid factor (RF) is detected in more than 80% of patients with rheumatoid arthritis and in up to 10% of patients with psoriatic arthritis [66], distinguishing psoriatic arthritis from rheumatoid arthritis can sometimes be challenging. Several clinical features independent of skin lesions help to distinguish the two diseases. Rheumatoid arthritis is more common in women, whereas psoriatic arthritis does not have a sex predilection. The joint distribution in psoriatic arthritis is such that all the joints of a single digit are more likely to be affected than the same joints on both sides as in patients with rheumatoid arthritis. The joint involvement in patients with rheumatoid arthritis tends to be more symmetrical. The DIP joints are uncommonly involved in patients with rheumatoid arthritis but frequently involved in patients with psoriatic arthritis. The joints of patients with psoriatic arthritis are less erythematous, less tender, and more fibrous than those in patients with rheumatoid arthritis. Rheumatoid nodules are absent in patients with psoriatic arthritis. Dactylitis is present in psoriatic arthritis but almost always absent in rheumatoid arthritis. Enthesitis is seen in 20–38% of psoriatic arthritis patients but almost always absent in rheumatoid arthritis [80, 90, 91].

Conclusions

Psoriasis is a common chronic recurrent inflammatory disease that can be disabling not only because of skin involvement but also because of concomitant joint disease. While the skin lesions are readily recognizable by the trained eye, psoriatic arthritis can sometimes be more difficult to diagnose. A broad base of knowledge of the clinical features and other disease associations of both psoriasis and psoriatic arthritis is important so that the most effective mode of therapy can be selected for these patients. As research into the etiology of psoriasis and the development of targeted immunotherapeutic agents to treat psoriasis and psoriatic arthritis continues, we will be able to advance the care of patients with these distressing and potentially disabling conditions.

References

1 Griffiths CEM, Christophers E, Barker JNWN, Chalmers RJG, Chimenti S, Krueger GG, Leonarid C, Menter A, Ortonne JP, Fry L (2007) A classification of psoriasis vulgaris according to phenotype. *Br J Dermatol* 156: 258–262

2 Biondi OC, Scarpa R, Pucino A, Oriente P (1989) Psoriasis and psoriatic arthritis. Dermatological and rheumatological co-operative clinical report. *Acta Dermatol Venereol* 146 (suppl): 69–71

3 McMillin BD, Maddern BR, Graham WR (1999) A role for tonsillectomy in the treatment of psoriasis? *Ear, Nose and Throat J* 78: 155–158

4 Boyd AS, Menter A (1989) Erythrodermic psoriasis: precipitating factors, course, and prognosis in 50 patients. *J Am Acad Dermatol* 21: 985–991

5 Farber EM, Nall ML (1974) The natural history of psoriasis in 5600 patients. *Dermatologica* 148: 1–18

6 Lewin K, De Wit S, Ferrington RA (1971) Nail involvement in psoriasis: a clinicopathological study. In: EM Farber, AJ Cox (eds): *Proceedings of the International Symposium on Psoriasis*, Stanford University Press, California, 111–123

7 Farber EM, Nall L (1992) Nail Psoriasis. *Cutis* 50: 174–178

8 Scher RK (1985) Psoriasis of the nail. *Dermatol Clinics* 3: 387–394

9 Hietanen J, Salo OP, Kanerva L, Juvakoski T (1984) Study of the oral mucosa in 200 consecutive patients. *Scand J Dent Res* 92: 50–54

10 Morris LF, Phillips CM, Binnie WH, Sander HM, Silverman AK, Menter MA (1992) Oral lesions in patients with psoriasis: a controlled study. *Cutis* 49: 339–344

11 Zhu JF, Kaminski MJ, Pulitzer DR, Hu J, Thomas HF (1996) Psoriasis: pathophysiology and oral manifestations. *Oral Dis* 2: 135–144

12 Yosipovitch G, Goon A, Wee J, Chan YH, Goh CL (2000) The prevalence and clinical characteristics of pruritus among patients with extensive psoriasis. *Br J Dermatol* 143: 969–973

13 Koo J (1996) Population-based epidemiologic study of psoriasis with emphasis on quality of life assessment. *Dermatol Clin* 14: 485–496

14 Szepietowski JC, Reich A, Wisnicka B (2004) Pruritus and psoriasis (letter). *Brit J Dermatol* 151: 1284

15 Krueger GG, Eyre RW (1984) Trigger factors in psoriasis. In: G Weinstein, MJ Voorhees (eds): *Dermatol Clin*. Philadelphia, Saunders, p. 373

16 Melski JW, Bernhard JD, Stern RS (1983) The Koebner (isomorphic) response in psoriasis: associations with early age of onset and multiple previous therapies. *Arch Dermatol* 19: 655–659

17 Nyfors A, Lemholt K (1975) Psoriasis in children: a short review and a survey of 245 cases. *Br J Dermatol* 92: 437–442

18 Whyte HJ, Baughman RD (1964) Acute guttate psoriasis and streptococcal infection. *Arch Dermatol* 89: 350–356

19 Telfer NR, Chalmers RJG, Whale K, Colman G (1992) The role of streptococcal infection in the

initiation of guttate psoriasis. *Arch Dermatol* 128: 39–42
20 Wilson JK, Al-Suwaidan SN, Krowchuk D, Feldman SR (2003) Treatment of psoriasis in children: is there a role for antibiotic therapy and tonsillectomy? *Ped Dermatol* 20: 11–15
21 Duvic M (1991) Papulosquamous disorders associated with human immunodeficiency virus infection. *Dermatol Clin* 9: 523–530
22 Mallon E, Bunker CB (2000) HIV-associated psoriasis. *AIDS Patient Care STDs* 14: 239–246
23 Colebunders R, Blot K, Meriens V, Dock P (1992) Psoriasis regression in terminal AIDS. *Lancet* 339: 1110
24 Johnson TM, Duvic M, Rapini RP, Rios A (1985) AIDS exacerbates psoriasis (letter). *N Engl J Med* 313: 1415
25 Fortune DG, Richards HL, Main CJ, Griffiths CE (1998) What patients with psoriasis believe about their condition. *J Am Acad Dermatol* 39: 196–201
26 Fortune DG, Richards HL, Kirby B, McElhone K, Markham T, Rogers S, Main CJ, Griffiths CE (2003) Psychological distress impairs clearance of psoriasis in patients treated with photochemotherapy. *Arch Dermatol* 139: 752–756
27 Fortune DG, Richards HL, Kirby B, Bowcock S, Main CJ, Griffiths CEM (2002) A cognitive-behavioural symptom management program as an adjunct in psoriasis therapy. *Br J Dermatol* 146: 458–465
28 Fortune DG, Richards HL, Griffiths CEM, Main CJ (2004) Targeting cognitive-behaviour therapy to patients' implicit model of psoriasis: results from a patient preference controlled trial. *Br J Clin Psychol* 43: 65–82
29 Tsankov N, Angelova I, Kazandjieva J (2000) Drug-induced psoriasis: recognition and management. *Am J Clin Dermatol* 1: 159–165
30 Higgins E (2000) Alcohol, smoking, and psoriasis. *Clin Exp Dermatol* 25: 107–110
31 Poikolainen K, Reunala T, Kiarvonen J, Lauharanta J, Karkkainen P (1990) Alcohol intake: a risk factor for psoriasis in young and middle aged men? *Br Med J* 300: 780–783
32 Poikolainen K, Reunala T, Karvonen J (1994) Smoking, alcohol and life events related to psoriasis among women. *Br J Dermatol* 130: 473–477
33 Duffy DL, Spelman LA, Martin NG (1993) Psoriasis in Australian twins. *J Am Acad Dermatol* 29: 428–434
34 Poikolainen K, Karvonen J, Pukkala E (1999) Excess mortality related to alcohol and smoking among hospital-treated patients with psoriasis. *Arch Dermatol* 135: 1490–1493
35 Herron MD, Hinckley M, Hoffman MS, Papenfuss J, Hansen CB, Callis KP, Krueger GG (2005) Impact of obesity and smoking on psoriasis presentation and management. *Arch Dermatol* 141: 1527–1534
36 Naldi L, Chatenoud L, Linder D, Belloni FA, Peserico A, Virgili AR, Bruni PL, Ingordo V, Lo Scocco G, Solaroli C et al. (2005) Cigarette smoking, body mass index, and stressful life events as risk factors for psoriasis: results from an Italian case-control study. *J Invest Dermatol* 125: 61–67
37 Fortes C, Mastroeni S, Leffondre K, Sampogna F, Melchi F, Mazzotti E, Pasquini P, Abeni D (2005) Relationship between smoking and the clinical severity of psoriasis. *Arch Dermatol* 141: 1580–1584
38 Mowad CM, Margolis DJ, Halpern AC, Suri B, Synnestvedt M, Guzzo CA (1998) Hormonal influences on women with psoriasis. *Cutis* 61: 257–260
39 Murase JE, Chan KK, Garite TJ, Cooper DM, Weinstein GD (2005) Hormonal effect on psoriasis in pregnancy and post partum. *Arch Dermatol* 141: 601–606
40 Boyd AS, Morris LF, Phillips CM, Menter MA (1996) Psoriasis and pregnancy: hormone and immune system interaction. *Int J Dermatol* 35: 169–172
41 Christensen TE, Callis KP, Papenfuss J, Hoffman MS, Hansen CB, Wong B, Panko JM, Krueger GG (2006) Observations of psoriasis in the absence of therapeutic intervention identifies two unappreciated morphologic variants, thin-plaque and thick-plaque psoriasis, and their associated phenotypes. *J Invest Dermatol* 126: 2397–2403
42 Johnson MT, Roberts J (1978) Skin conditions and related need for medical care among persons 1–74 years. *Vital Health Stat* 11: 1–72
43 Naldi L (2004) Epidemiology of psoriasis. *Curr Drug Targets Inflamm Allergy* 3: 121–128
44 Lebwohl M (2003) Psoriasis. *Lancet* 361: 1197–1204
45 Kenney JA (1965) Management of dermatoses peculiar to Negroes. *Arch Dermatol* 91: 126–129
46 Gelfand JM, Stern RS, Nijsten T, Feldman SR, Thomas J, Kist J, Rolstad T, Margolis DJ (2005)

The prevalence of psoriasis in African Americans: results from a population-based study. *J Am Acad Dermatol* 52: 23–26
47 Lomholt G (1971) Psoriasis in Uganda: A comparative study with other parts of Africa. In: EM Farber, AJ Cox (eds): *Proceedings of the International Symposium on Psoriasis*. Stanford University Press, California, 41–48
48 Schon MP, Boehncke WH (2005) Medical progress: Psoriasis. *N Engl J Med* 352: 1899–1912
49 Buntin D, Skinner R, Rosenberg E (1983) Onset of psoriasis at age 108. *J Am Acad Dermatol* 9: 276–277
50 Holgate MC (1975) The age-of-onset of psoriasis and the relationship to parental psoriasis. *Br J Dermatol* 92: 443–448
51 Ferrandiz C, Pujol RM, Garcia-Patos V, Bordas X, Smandia JA (2002) Psoriasis of early and late onset: a clinical and epidemiologic study from Spain. *J Am Acad Dermatol* 46: 867–873
52 Farber EM, Nall ML (1971) Genetics of psoriasis: Twin study. In: EM Farber, AJ Cox (eds): *Proceedings of the International Symposium on Psoriasis*. Stanford University Press, California, 7–13
53 Henseler T, Christophers E (1985) Psoriasis of early and late onset: characterizations of two types of psoriasis vulgaris. *J Am Acad Dermatol* 13: 450–456
54 Yates VM, Watkinson G, Kelman A (1982) Further evidence for an association between psoriasis, Crohn's disease and ulcerative colitis. *Br J Dermatol* 106: 323–330
55 Najarian DJ, Gottlieb AB (2003) Connections between psoriasis and Crohn's disease. *J Am Acad Dermatol* 48: 805–821
56 Mallbris L, Granath F, Hamsten A, Stahle M (2006) Psoriasis is associated with lipid abnormalities at the onset of skin disease. *J Am Acad Dermatol* 54: 614–621
57 Naldi L, Parazzini F, Peli L, Chatenoud L, Cainelli T (1996) Dietary factors and the risk of psoriasis. Results of an Italian case-control study. *Br J Dermatol* 134: 101–106
58 Neimann AL, Shin DB, Wang X, Margolis DJ, Troxel AB, Gelfand JM (2006) Prevalence of cardiovascular risk factors in patients with psoriasis. *J Am Acad Dermatol* 55: 829–835
59 Gelfand JM, Neimann AL, Shin DB, Wang X, Margolis DJ, Troxel AB (2006) Risk of myocardial infarction in patients with psoriasis. *J Am Med Assoc* 296: 1735–1741
60 Shapiro J, Cohen AD, David M, Hodak E, Chodik G, Viner A, Kremer E, Heymann A (2007) The association between psoriasis, diabetes mellitus, and atherosclerosis in Israel: A case-control study. *J Am Acad Dermatol* 56: 629–634
61 Sommer DM, Jenisch S, Suchan M, Christophers E, Weichenthal M (2006) Increased prevalence of the metabolic syndrome in patients with moderate to severe psoriasis. *Arch Dermatol Res* 298: 321–328
62 Zachariae N, Sogaard H (1973) Liver biopsy in psoriasis. A controlled study. *Dermatologica* 146: 149–155
63 Christophers E (2001) Psoriasis – epidemiology and clinical spectrum. *Clin Exp Dermatol* 26: 314–320
64 Gelfand JM, Berlin J, Van Voorhees A, Margolis DJ (2003) Lymphoma rates are low but increased in patients with psoriasis: results from a population-based cohort study in the United Kingdom. *Arch Dermatol* 139: 1425–1429
65 Gelfand JM, Shin DB, Neimann AL, Xingmei Wang, Margolis DJ, Troxel AB (2006) The risk of lymphoma in patients with psoriasis. *J Invest Dermatol* 126: 2194–2201
66 Moll JM, Wright V (1973) Psoriatic Arthritis. *Semin Arthritis Rheum* 3: 55–78
67 Gladman DD, Atoni C, Mease P, Clegg DO, Nash P (2005) Psoriatic arthritis: epidemiology, clinical features, course, and outcome. *Ann Rheum Dis* 64 (suppl II): ii14–ii17
68 Gladman DD (2002) Current concepts in psoriatic arthritis. *Curr Opin Rheumatol* 14: 361–366
69 Gladman DD (1995) Psoriatic arthritis. *Baillieres Clin Rheumatol* 9: 319–329
70 Boumpas DT, Tassiulas IO (1997) Psoriatic arthritis. In: JH Klippel (ed.): *Primer of the Rheumatic Diseases*. Arthritis Foundation, Atlanta, 175–179
71 Gladman DD, Shuckett R, Russell ML, Thorne JC, Schachter RK (1987) Psoriatic arthritis (PSA) – An analysis of 220 patients. *Quart J Med* 62: 127–141
72 Moul DK, Korman NJ (2005) The early signs and symptoms of psoriatic arthritis: the importance of early evaluation and treatment. *Psoriasis Forum* 11: 4–6
73 Goupille P, Laulan J, Vedere V, Kaplan G, Valat JP (1995) Psoriatic onycho-periostitis. Report of three cases. *Scand J Rheumatol* 24: 53–54
74 Siannis F, Farewell V, Cook R, Schentag C, Gladman D (2006) Clinical and radiological damage

in psoriatic arthritis. *Ann Rheum Dis* 65: 478–481
75 Johnson SR, Schentag CT, Gladman DD (2005) Autoantibodies in biological agent naïve patients with psoriatic arthritis. *Ann Rheum Dis* 64: 770–772
76 Cruyssen VB, Hoffman IE, Zmierczak H, Van den Berghe M, Kruithof E, De Rycke L, Mielants H, Veys EM, Baeten D, De Keyser F (2005) Anti-citrullinated peptide antibodies may occur in patients with psoriatic arthritis. *Ann Rheum Dis* 64:1145–1149
77 Bogliolo L, Alpini C, Caporali R, Scire CA, Moratti R, Montecucco C (2005) Antibodies to cyclic citrullinated peptides in psoriatic arthritis. *J Rheumatol* 32: 511–515
78 Gladman DD (1998) Clinical aspects of the spondyloarthropathies. *Am J Med Sci* 316: 234–238
79 Gladman DD, Anhorn KA, Schachter RK, Mervart H (1986) HLA antigens in psoriatic arthritis. *J Rheumatol* 13: 586–592
80 Gladman DD (1994) The natural history of psoriatic arthritis. In: V Wright, PS Helliwel (eds): *Bailliere's Clinical Rheumatology. International Practice and Research.* Bailliere Tindall, London, 379–394
81 Kane D, Stafford L, Bresnihan B, FitzGerald O (2003) A prospective, clinical and radiological study of early psoriatic arthritis: an early synovitis clinic experience. *Rheumatology* 42: 1460–1468
82 Buskila D, Langevitz P, Gladman DD, Urowitz S, Smythe HA (1992) Patients with rheumatoid arthritis are more tender than those with psoriatic arthritis. *J Rheumatol* 19: 1115–1119
83 Cantini F, Salvarani C, Olivieri I, Macchioni L, Miccoli L, Padula A, Falcone C, Boiardi L, Bozza A, Barozzi L et al. (2001) Distal extremity swelling with pitting edema in psoriatic arthritis: a case-control study. *Clin Exp Rheumatol* 19: 291–296
84 Jones SM, Armas JB, Cohen MG, Lovell CR, Evison G, McHugh NJ (1994) Psoriatic arthritis: outcome of disease subsets and relationship of joint disease to nail and skin disease. *Br J Rheumatol* 33: 834–839
85 Shbeeb M, Uramoto KM, Gibson LE, O'Fallon WM, Gabriel SE (2000) The epidemiology of psoriatic arthritis in Olmsted County, Minnesota, USA, 1982–1991. *J Rheumatol* 27: 1247–1250
86 Gelfand JM, Gladman DD, Mease PJ, Smith N, Margolis DJ, Nijsten T, Stern RS, Feldman SR, Rolstad T (2005) Epidemiology of psoriatic arthritis in the population of the United States. *J Am Acad Dermatol* 53: 573–577
87 Brockbank J, Gladman D (2002) Diagnosis and management of psoriatic arthritis. *Drugs* 62: 2447–2460
88 Madland TM, Apalset EM, Johannessen AE, Rossebo B, Brun JG (2005) Prevalence, disease manifestations, and treatment of psoriatic arthritis in Western Norway. *J Rheumatol* 32: 1918–1922
89 Williamson L, Dalbeth N, Dockerty JL, Gee BC, Weatherall R, Wordsworth BP (2004) Extended report: nail disease in psoriatic arthritis – clinically important, potentially treatable and often overlooked. *Rheumatology* 43: 790–794
90 Lavaroni G, Kokelj F, Pauluzzi P, Trevisan G (1994) The nails in psoriatic arthritis. *Acta Derm Venereol* 186 (suppl): 113
91 Oriente P, Biondi-Oriente C, Scarpa R (1994) Psoriatic arthritis: clinical manifestations. *Bailleres Clin Rheumatol* 8: 277–294

Treatment of Psoriasis
Edited by J.M. Weinberg

Topical therapy I: corticosteroids and vitamin D analogs

Paru R. Chaudhari, Dana K. Stern and Mark G. Lebwohl

Mount Sinai School of Medicine Department of Dermatology, 5 E 98th St 5th Floor, New York, NY 10029, USA

Introduction

Topical therapy is the first-line of treatment for mild to moderate psoriasis (see Tab. 1). The following two chapters will describe the available topical therapies for psoriasis, providing insight into the progress that has been made for treatment of the disease. This chapter will focus on the most widely used topical regimens, topical corticosteroids and vitamin D analogs, while the subsequent chapter will examine additional topical therapies used to treat psoriasis.

Table 1. Topical psoriasis treatments

Anthralin
Corticosteroids
Salicylic acid
Tar
Tazarotene
Topical immunomodulators
Vitamin D analogs

Topical corticosteroids

Mechanism of action

Topical corticosteroid therapy for inflammatory skin diseases was first introduced in 1952 and remains a mainstay of modern therapy [1]. Steroids are therapeutic by virtue of their anti-inflammatory, antiproliferative, immunosuppressive and vasoconstrictive properties [2]. They bind to cellular steroid-receptors to form a steroid-receptor complex, which is then transported into the cell nucleus to attach to glucocorticoid-response elements (GRE) on DNA. Attachment to GRE by the complex results in stimulation or inhibition of gene transcription, which can regulate the inflammatory processes that occur in psoriasis. Steroids can also affect transcription of genes that do not contain GRE receptors by inhibiting nuclear factor-κB (NF-κB), a factor that increases proinflammatory cytokines that normally contribute to psoriatic lesions. This inhibition of NF-κB occurs with corticosteroid stimulation of the inhibitory nuclear factor κBα (IκBα) [3, 4]. The resulting changes in gene transcription by GRE and non-GRE methods alter proinflammatory cytokines, such as interleukin (IL)-1, IL-2, IL-6, interferon gamma, and tumor necrosis factor-alpha [5]. By decreasing these cytokines, steroids directly contribute to the inhibition of capillary dilation, vascular permeability and dermal edema, along with the suppression of endothelial cell and lymphocyte activity normally seen in psoriasis [2].

Adverse effects

Side effects of topical corticosteroids include both local and systemic reactions (see Tab. 2). Local cutaneous side effects are common at steroid-sensitive sites, such as the face and intertriginous areas, or at any location subjected to long-term use. The face is a steroid-sensitive site due its relatively thin skin, while intertriginous areas are sensitive due to their tendency to self-occlude. Topical corticosteroids can cause atrophy of the epidermis and dermis leaving thin, fragile skin, with visible telangiectases. Even minor trauma on this delicate skin can lead to breakage of small vessels as well as purpura [6]. Atrophy begins as early as three days at any location receiving topical corticosteroids,

Table 2. Topical corticosteroid side effects

Local	Bruising
	Changes in pigmentation
	Hirsutism
	Perioral dermatitis
	Purpura
	Rebound Flare
	Steroid atrophy
	Steroid Rosacea
	Striae
	Telangiectases
	Ulcers
Systemic	Bilateral femoral avascular necrosis
	Cataracts
	Endocrine, metabolic, electrolytic effects
	Glaucoma
	Growth retardation
	Hypothalamic-pituitary-adrenal axis suppression
Tachyphylaxis	

due to a decline in cell size and number of layers in the epidermis [2]. In addition, irreversible striae can occur as a result of damage to dermal connective tissue [7]. These dermal changes are attributed to a decrease of collagen and mucopolysaccharides as a result of the antiproliferative effect of corticosteroids on fibroblasts [6].

Systemic effects, although infrequent, are more often noted in patients treated with high potency corticosteroids due to an increased concentration of steroid absorbed into the blood stream. In general, these systemic adverse events occur when steroids are used for prolonged periods of time or at doses higher than commonly prescribed. An uncommon, yet serious, systemic side effect is hypothalamic-pituitary-adrenal axis suppression, which has been seen after the use of both medium-potency and superpotent topical corticosteroids [7]. There have even been reported deaths secondary to use of topical corticosteroids at high doses; in one case, a patient had been applying over 200 g of clobetasol propionate per week in addition to other topical corticosteroids for many years [8]. Other rare, systemic side effects include Cushing syndrome and bilateral femoral avascular necrosis [9–12]. Topical steroids applied to the periorbital region can lead to glaucoma and therefore caution must be used when prescribing potent steroids to this area [13]. Topical corticosteroids should not be applied to greater than 20% body surface area due to the risk of increased systemic absorption and side effects. In addition, superpotent corticosteroids should not be used continuously for greater than 2–4 weeks.

Tachyphylaxis, where corticosteroids have diminished efficacy after repeated use, is another side effect of topical corticosteroid therapy [14]. Miller et al. questioned the existence of tachyphylaxis. More than half of the clinical dermatologists surveyed in this study believed in the existence of tachyphylaxis, but a clinical trial failed to demonstrate the phenomenon [15]. Some attribute the apparent tachyphylaxis to lack of patient adherence to tedious corticosteroid regimens, while others believe that there is actually a sudden worsening of psoriasis or persistence of underlying disease unrelated to the effectiveness of the corticosteroids [6, 16].

Topical corticosteroids use in pregnancy and in pediatric populations

Although psoriasis has been reported to improve during pregnancy, many patients still require topical therapy throughout their pregnancy. Safety concerns for the developing fetus must be considered, however [17]. Topical corticosteroids are labeled as category C (see Tab. 3) and are prescribed as treatment if the benefits of therapy outweigh the risks. Although topical corticosteroids are prescribed during pregnancy and considered relatively safe with few reported adverse events, one case report attributed intrauterine growth retardation to the use of 40 mg/day of topical triamcinolone during the 12th week of gestation [18].

Table 3. Categories for drug use during pregnancy

Category A	Adequate and well-controlled studies have failed to demonstrate a risk to the fetus in the first trimester of pregnancy (and there is no evidence of risk in later trimesters).
Category B	Animal reproduction studies have failed to demonstrate a risk to the fetus and there are no adequate and well-controlled studies in pregnant women OR animal studies have shown an adverse effect, but adequate and well-controlled studies in pregnant women have failed to demonstrate a risk to the fetus in any trimester.
Category C	Animal reproduction studies have shown an adverse effect on the fetus and there are no adequate and well-controlled studies in humans, but potential benefits may warrant use of the drug in pregnant women despite potential risks
Category D	There is positive evidence of human fetal risk based on adverse reaction data from investigational or marketing experience or studies in humans, but potential benefits may warrant use of the drug in pregnant women despite potential risks.
Category X	Studies in animals or humans have demonstrated fetal abnormalities and/or there is positive evidence of human fetal risk based on adverse reaction data from investigational or marketing experience, and the risks involved in use of the drug in pregnant women clearly outweigh potential benefits.

Reprinted from http://www.fda.gov/fdac/features/2001/301_preg.html#categories

Infants and younger children are at greater risk for side effects due to their higher skin surface-to-body mass ratio, which is approximately 2.5 to 3 times that of adults. Both growth retardation and suppression of the HPA axis have been documented in children more frequently than in older populations [19–21]. As a result of increased systemic absorption, children need to be monitored more conservatively. Use of superpotent agents should be limited to short periods of time when necessary [22].

Therapeutic response

Topical corticosteroids are ranked in potency based on their ability to vasoconstrict, described by the Stoughton-Cornell classification system in 1985 [23]. They range from Class 1 (superpotent) to Class 7 (available as over the counter drugs) (Tab. 4). Regimens are tailored to maintain efficacy while minimizing local and systemic side effects. Class 1 therapies should not be used continuously for longer than 2 weeks and, once lesions are under control, maintenance therapy can include a lower potency drug or intermittent use of a superpotent therapy (e.g., weekend therapy) [24]. In children with atopic eczema, brief treatment with a potent topical corticosteroid was equivalent in efficacy to prolonged treatment with mild corticosteroids during a double blind, randomized 18-week study [25]. Similarly, a study using twice-daily fluticasone propionate ointment 0.005% for 2 weeks followed by once-daily application on two consecutive days for 8 weeks resulted in rapid healing of psoriasis and a reduced local side effect profile [26].

Low potency corticosteroids are used more often on sensitive areas such as the face, groin, and axilla, while thick, chronic plaques are treated with high-

Table 4. Corticosteroid potency

Class 1 – Superpotent	Betamethasone dipropionate 0.05% gel/ointment Clobetasol propionate 0.05% cream/ointment/lotion Diflorasone diacetate 0.05% ointment Halobetasol propionate 0.05% cream/ointment Fluocinonide 0.1% cream
Class 2 – Potent	Amcinonide 0.1% ointment Betamethasone dipropionate 0.05% ointment Desoximetasone 0.25%/0.05% cream/ointment Fluocinonide 0.05% cream/ointment Halcinonide 0.1% cream
Class 3 – Upper midstrength	Betamethasone dipropionate 0.05% cream Betamethasone valerate 0.1% ointment Fluticasone propionate 0.005% ointment Mometasone furoate 0.1% ointment Triamcinolone acetonide 0.5% cream
Class 4 – Midstrength	Betamethasone valerate 0.12% foam Clocortolone pivalate 0.1% cream Desoximetasone 0.05% cream Fluocinolone acetonide 0.2% cream/ointment Flurandrenolide 0.05% ointment Triamcinolone acetonide 0.1% cream/ointment
Class 5 – Lower mid-strength	Betamethasone dipropionate 0.05% lotion Betamethasone valerate 0.1% cream/lotion Fluocinolone acetonide 0.025% cream Flurandrenolide 0.05% cream Fluticasone propionate 0.05% cream Hydrocortisone butyrate 0.1% cream Hydrocortisone valerate 0.2% cream Prednicarbate 0.1% cream Triamcinolone acetonide 0.1% cream/lotion
Class 6 – Mild strength	Alclometasone dipropionate 0.05% cream/ointment Desonide 0.05% cream Fluocinolone acetonide 0.01% cream/solution
Class 7 – Least potent	Topicals with hydrocortisone, dexamethasone, flumethasone, methylprednisolone, and prednisolon

Adapted from Del Rosso J, Friedlander SF (2005) Corticosteroids: Options in the era of steroid-sparing therapy. *J Am Acad Dermatol* 53: S50–58

er-potency agents [27]. Intertriginous areas tend to self-occlude and therefore lower potency therapy is needed. Due to the number of topical corticosteroids available, risk/benefit ratios have been analyzed to determine the therapies that cause the least amount of side effects in each potency class. These studies suggest that fluticasone propionate [26], mometasone furoate [28], prednicarbate and tipredane [29, 30] have a favorable risk/benefit ratio [7]. However, other topical corticosteroids have not been studied as closely as the aforementioned drugs.

Corticosteroids are available in different vehicles including lotions, solutions, creams, ointment, gels, sprays, tapes, and foams [31]. The vehicles differ in action and potency and are often chosen based on the portion of the body affected by psoriasis. Glabrous areas, such as the palms and soles, along with the trunk and extremities are often treated with ointments, while foams and gels are used more in hairy and oily areas [2]. Novel foam vehicles of mid-potency betamethasone valerate (BMV) and ultra-high-potency clobetasol propionate (CP) were found to be safe and effective with rapid absorption and better compliance, including in the difficult-to-treat scalp region, shown in multiple clinical trials [32–34].

Topical corticosteroids as combination therapy

Topical corticosteroids are commonly used in conjunction with other topical treatments or ultraviolet (UV) light for treatment of psoriasis in order to maximize efficacy and minimize side effects [35]. Combination therapy, where two or more drugs are used concurrently, leads to a synergistic response at lower doses than either therapy alone. Because corticosteroids are commonly combined with other topical therapies, these regimens will be reviewed during our discussion of vitamin D analogs and in the following chapter.

Topical corticosteroids combined with either ultraviolet B (UVB) or psoralen plus ultraviolet A (PUVA) have been studied as possible psoriasis therapy. No improvement in psoriasis was noted with the combination of UVB and topical corticosteroids; in fact, combination therapy may actually shorten remission time [36]. In contrast, when PUVA is combined with topical corticosteroids, it leads to rapid clearance of psoriatic lesions at a lower cumulative UVA dose, making it an advantageous regimen [35]. The results on remission time are less clear; some argue that the PUVA/topical corticosteroid combination rapidly clears the disease without altering remission time, while others conclude that remission is actually shortened [37, 38].

Topical vitamin D analogs

Mechanism of action

Calcipotriol (calcipotriene in the US), a vitamin D_3 analog, was first introduced as topical treatment for psoriasis in the early 1990s. Efficacy of vitamin D was first suggested when Morimoto and Kumahara reported drastic improvement of psoriasis in a patient taking oral vitamin D [39]. Along with intestinal calcium absorption and bone mineralization, Vitamin D_3 can inhibit cellular proliferation and stimulate cellular differentiation [40]. The inhibition of cellular proliferation and stimulation of differentiation was also noted in keratinocytes, thus supporting the idea for use as a psoriasis therapy [41]. Because of the potential effects of vitamin D_3, activated as 1, 25-dihydroxyvitamin D_3, on serum calcium levels, analogs were created as topical treatments. Since then, vitamin D_3 analogs have become a mainstay in the dermatologic treatment of psoriasis.

Calcipotriol, similar to 1, 25-dihydroxyvitamin D_3 but 200 times less likely to cause hypercalcemia, binds to intracellular vitamin D receptors (VDR). The resulting complex interacts with regions of DNA known as the vitamin D response element (VDRE) [42, 43]. This interaction leads to transcriptional changes that have multiple effects including inhibition of phosphorylation of epidermal growth factor (EGF) receptors in a calcium-dependent manner [44, 45]. Deactivation of EGF may be responsible for the ability of topical vitamin D analogs to inhibit cellular proliferation and stimulate cellular differentiation [46]. Topical vitamin D analogs are also able to alter inflammatory responses. In summary, it is the inhibition of cellular proliferation and stimulation of cellular differentiation that greatly contribute to the therapeutic benefit of vitamin D analogs on psoriasis.

Adverse effects

Patients on topical vitamin D therapy are at risk for local and, rarely, systemic side effects. Local side effects such as irritation occur in as many as 20% of patients treated with calcipotriol ointment, especially in sensitive areas like the face. Irritation usually develops within the first few weeks of treatment and remains stable throughout the course of therapy [47, 48]. Calcitriol ointment tends to cause less irritation than calcipotriol ointment [49]. Topical tacalcitol, a more recent vitamin D analog, is also more tolerable in sensitive areas [50].

Systemic alterations in calcium homeostasis and bone metabolism are theoretical concerns associated with vitamin D therapy; however, several studies have failed to demonstrate these adverse affects. In a double-blind randomized trial looking at the short-term effects of calcipotriol *versus* placebo, no differences were found in bone and calcium metabolism [51]. The cumulative effect of long-term vitamin D analog therapy on serum calcium levels is also of concern, but serum and urinary calcium remained stable even after a year of 30 g per week of calcipotriol [52]. Statistically significant changes in serum parathyroid hormone and urinary calcium, however, occurred when patients were exposed to 100 g/week of calcipotriol [52–54]. Patients with renal impairment need to be observed carefully since there have been reported cases of hypercalcemia in patients receiving doses less than 100 g/week [55, 56]. Hypercalcemia was also noted in a patient taking both tacalcitol and a thiazide diuretic, a drug that may enhance serum calcium [57]. Vitamin D therapy is contraindicated in patients already suffering from hypercalcemia.

Topical vitamin D analog use in pregnancy and pediatric populations

Vitamin D analogs have not been found to be teratogenic in animals, although no clinical data on humans has been reported. Treatment with vitamin D analogs during pregnancy is rated Category C (Tab. 3) [58]. Use of calcipotriol for the treatment of psoriasis in children is effective, with minor skin irritation and no metabolic effects at rates up to 50 g/week [59, 60].

Therapeutic response

Because of the side effects of topical corticosteroids, steroid-sparing agents such as vitamin D analogs are an exciting addition to the armamentarium of topical therapy. The therapeutic benefits of calcitriol, calcipotriol (calcipotriene), and the newer vitamin D analogs such as tacalcitol, have been examined in numerous clinical trials for over a decade. During the first double-blind study using calcipotriol cream, patients showed significant improvement in psoriatic lesions, both scaling and erythema, and minimal adverse effects [61]. Further studies concluded that twice-daily calcipotriol 0.005% ointment was the ideal therapeutic dose, and in one double-blind, right-left comparison trial, 74.2% of patients showed significant improvement of psoriatic lesions after 4 weeks of treatment. Calcipotriol does display a slower onset of action, however, than other topical therapies [62–64].

The efficacy of calcipotriol ointment is equivalent to Class 2 corticosteroids for treatment of plaque psoriasis [65]. In comparison to superpotent topical corticosteroids, vitamin D analogs have delayed clinical onset but result in longer disease-free periods. In a randomized, double-blind, 8 week study, 48% of patients on vitamin D therapy remained in remission compared to only 25% on betamethasone therapy [66]. Another study demonstrated that calcipotriol has equivalent efficacy to anthralin, a traditional topical therapy, but patients preferred the vitamin D analog because of its more tolerable side effect profile [67]. Newer vehicles of calcipotriol have also been developed to treat psoriasis in difficult-to-treat areas. For example, a calcipotriol solution has been produced for scalp psoriasis, and a study with over 3'000 patients found it both effective and well-tolerated [68].

Calcitriol, available in Europe, is also effective for the treatment of psoriasis, especially on sensitive areas of the skin [69]. Because calcipotriol often causes irritation on the face and in intertriginous sites, calcitriol is a valuable alternative for psoriasis in these areas. Calcitriol may have greater effects on serum calcium, however, in comparison to the analogs [49]. Another vitamin D analog, tacalcitol, inhibits keratinocyte proliferation and stimulates differentiation and has equivalent potency to calcipotriol [70]. Tacalcitol was originally approved for psoriasis in Japan as a twice a day 2 μg/g regimen and later in Europe as a once-a-day 4 μg/g treatment. Clinical studies done by Van De Kerkhof et al. have shown tacalcitol ointment to be a safe and effective long-term treatment for psoriasis with rare systemic side effects and good tolerability in sensitive areas [50, 71]. Direct comparison of twice-a-day calcipotriol and once-a-day tacalcitol during a double-blind trial by Veien et al. demonstrated, however, a therapeutic advantage for calcipotriol after 8 weeks of treatment on psoriatic plaques [72]. New vitamin D analogs are currently under investigation for the treatment of psoriasis. Maxacalcitol has recently been found effective, but additional clinical studies are necessary [73]. A pilot study for paricalcitol, a vitamin D analog developed for the prevention of secondary hyperparathyroidism, has also shown positive results for the treatment of psoriasis [74].

Topical vitamin D analogs as combination therapy

Topical vitamin D analogs have been effectively combined with other topical therapy, UV light and systemic therapy for the treatment of psoriasis. Multiple clinical trials have demonstrated therapeutic benefits when topical vitamin D analogs are used in combination with topical corticosteroids. One multicenter trial showed that once-daily halobetasol propionate 0.005% ointment with once-daily calcipotriol was more effective than either treatment as monotherapy at treating psoriatic lesions [75]. In this study, 71% of patients treated with calcipotriol/halobetasol were clear or almost clear compared to 30% in the calcipotriol group and 57% in the halobetasol group after 14 days of treatment. Another study investigating the vitamin D/corticosteroid combination as a maintenance regimen concluded that twice-daily halobetasol ointment on weekends and calcipotriol ointment on weekdays was significantly better than twice-daily halobetasol ointment alone on weekends. 76% of patients applying the combination remained in remission for 6 months as opposed to 40% of patients applying halobetasol ointment alone [76]. This combination not only improved psoriatic lesions, but also limited the atrophic side effects of corticosteroids. As a result of these studies, topical vitamin D analogs and corticosteroids are commonly prescribed together for the treatment of psoriasis.

Calcipotriol and betamethasone dipropionate are now available in a single ointment. For the past several years, multiple studies have shown the safety and efficacy of the two-compound treatment for psoriasis [77–80]. In an 8 week, randomized, double-blind, vehicle-controlled trial with 1'106 patients, the combination of calcipotriol and betamethosone dipropionate doubled PASI reduction in comparison to either treatment as monotherapy [77]. The two-compound treatment also displays a rapid onset of action and fewer adverse events. Within the first week of treatment, Papp et al. showed that calcipotriol/betamethasone dipropionate significantly reduced the mean percentage of PASI in comparison to steroid monotherapy [78]. Further, the two-compound product had a significantly decreased local side effect profile compared to calcipotriol alone after 12 weeks of therapy [81]. In another double-blind, randomized, vehicle-controlled trial, Guenther et al. showed that the two-compound product is safe and effective when used twice-daily [79]. The combined product is also effective when used for lengthier time periods. A recent 52-week, randomized, double-blind study with over 600 patients showed that the two-compound treatment once-daily remained efficacious and had limited side effects over that period of time [82, 83]. Calcipotriol/betamethosone dipropionate has been studied as a maintenance regimen as well. In a randomized, parallel-group clinical trial, 4 weeks of treatment with the two-compound product followed by 8 weeks of calcipotriol cream on weekdays and the two-compound product on weekends was an effective treatment for psoriasis [84]. A recent comparison of six Phase III trials found that the combination of calcipotriol and betamethasone dipropionate consistently provided rapid and highly effective therapy for psoriasis [85]. Foam vehicles for topical corticosteroids have also sparked new combination and maintenance therapies. CP foam followed by calcipotriol ointment is more effective than either agent alone [86]. Additionally, twice-daily CP foam on weekends with twice-daily calcipotriol on weekdays led to 92% clearance of psoriatic trunk lesions compared to only 62% with calcipotriol and vehicle after 6 months of treatment [87].

During a 2-week pilot study, calcipotriol ointment combined with tazarotene gel cleared psoriatic plaques as effectively as a Class 1 topical corticosteroid [88]. Further trials are necessary to confirm that these steroid-sparing agents combined are more effective than their individual therapies. Because calcipotriol is an easily degraded molecule, combination with topical treatments for psoriasis is not always an option. 6% salicylic acid, hydrocortisone 17-valerate and 12% ammonium lactate all inactivate the vitamin D analog [89].

Results of studies combining calcipotriol and UV therapy are mixed [35]. Although many initial trials suggested that calcipotriol enhances the effect of UVB as treatment for psoriasis, a meta-analysis done in 2000 demonstrated no difference between UVB/calcipotriol and UVB alone or calcipotriol alone [90–94]. Narrowband UVB (NBUVB) plus calcipotriol was also found to be equivalent to NBUVB alone for the treatment of psoriasis [95]. In contrast, the combination of PUVA and calcipotriol has been found to be an effective treatment for psoriasis. The first study that looked at calcipotriol/PUVA took place in 1993 and multiple subsequent studies have demonstrated that the combination leads to rapid improvement of psoriasis at a lower cumulative dose of UVA [7, 35, 96]. Because UVA inactivates the vitamin D analog, it is important to apply calcipotriol after light therapy [97].

The systemic agents, acitretin, methotrexate and cyclosporine, have all been successfully combined with topical vitamin D analogs. A double-blind randomized control trial found that topical calcipotriol plus oral acitretin was not only more effective at treating psoriasis, but the combination also allowed for a significantly lower cumulative dose of acitretin [98]. These findings were corroborated in a meta-analysis of calcipotriol combination therapies [90]. Methotrexate and calcipotriol share similar results, with significant improvement of psoriasis at a lower cumulative dose of methotrexate [99]. Low-dose cyclosporine and calcipotriol are also more successful for the treatment of psoriasis than either treatment as monotherapy. In a multicenter, placebo-controlled study, clearance occurred in almost 50% of patients with severe disease with the combined regimen in contrast to only 11.8% with 2 mg/kg/day cyclosporine alone [100].

References

1 Sulzberger MB, Witten VH (1952) The effect of topically applied compound F in selected dermatoses. *J Invest Dermatol* 19: 101–102

2 Hughes J, Rustin M (1997) Corticosteroids. *Clin Dermatol* 15: 715–721

3 Scheinman RI, Cogswell PC, Lofquist AK, Baldwin AS Jr, (1995) Role of transcriptional activation of I kappa B alpha in mediation of immunosuppression by glucocorticoids. *Science* 270: 283–286

4 Auphan N, DiDonato JA, Rosette C, Helmberg A, Karin M (1995) Immunosuppression by glucocorticoids: inhibition of NF-kappa B activity through induction of I kappa B synthesis. *Science* 270: 286–290

5 Almawi WY, Lipman ML, Stevens AC, Zanker B, Hadro ET, Strom TB (1991) Abrogation of glucocorticoid-mediated inhibition of T cell proliferation by the synergistic action of IL-1, IL-6, and IFN-gamma. *J Immunol* 146: 3523–3527

6 Del Rosso J, Friedlander SF (2005) Corticosteroids: options in the era of steroid-sparing therapy. *J Am Acad Dermatol* 53: S50–58

7 Lebwohl M, Ali S (2001) Treatment of psoriasis. Part 1. Topical therapy and phototherapy. *J Am Acad Dermatol* 45: 487–498; quiz 499–502

8 Nathan AW, Rose GL (1979) Fatal iatrogenic Cushing's syndrome. *Lancet* 1: 207

9 Reichert-Penetrat S, Trechot P, Barbaud A, Gillet P, Schmutz JL (2001) Bilateral femoral avascular necrosis in a man with psoriasis: responsibility of topical corticosteroids and role of cyclosporine. *Dermatology* 203: 356–357

10 Kane D, Barnes L, Fitzgerald O (2003) Topical corticosteroid treatment: systemic side-effects. *Br J Dermatol* 149: 417

11 Gilbertson EO, Spellman MC, Piacquadio DJ, Mulford MI (1998) Super potent topical corticosteroid use associated with adrenal suppression: clinical considerations. *J Am Acad Dermatol* 38: 318–321

12 Ermis B, Ors R, Tastekin A, Ozkan B (2003) Cushing's syndrome secondary to topical corticosteroids abuse. *Clin Endocrinol (Oxf)* 58: 795–796

13 Nielsen NV, Sorensen PN (1978) Glaucoma induced by application of corticosteroids to the periorbital region. *Arch Dermatol* 114: 953–954

14 du Vivier A, Stoughton RB (1975) Tachyphylaxis to the action of topically applied corticosteroids. *Arch Dermatol* 111: 581–583

15 Miller JJ, Roling D, Margolis D, Guzzo C (1999) Failure to demonstrate therapeutic tachyphylaxis to topically applied steroids in patients with psoriasis. *J Am Acad Dermatol* 41: 546–549

16 Feldman SR (2006) Tachyphylaxis to topical corticosteroids: the more you use them, the less they work? *Clin Dermatol* 24: 229–230; discussion 230

17 Dunna SF, Finlay AY (1989) Psoriasis: improvement during and worsening after pregnancy. *Br J Dermatol* 120: 584

18 Katz VL, Thorp JM Jr, Bowes WA Jr, (1990) Severe symmetric intrauterine growth retardation associated with the topical use of triamcinolone. *Am J Obstet Gynecol* 162: 396–397

19 Turpeinen M, Salo OP, Leisti S (1986) Effect of percutaneous absorption of hydrocortisone on adrenocortical responsiveness in infants with severe skin disease. *Br J Dermatol* 115: 475–484

20 Lucky AW, Grote GD, Williams JL, Tuley MR, Czernielewski JM, Dolak TM, Herndon JH, Baker MD (1997) Effect of desonide ointment, 0.05%, on the hypothalamic-pituitary-adrenal axis of children with atopic dermatitis. *Cutis* 59: 151–153

21 Vermeer BJ, Heremans GF (1974) A case of growth retardation and cushing's syndrome due to

excessive application of betamethasone-17-valerate ointment. *Dermatologica* 149: 299–304
22 Hengge UR, Ruzicka T, Schwartz RA, Cork MJ (2006) Adverse effects of topical glucocorticosteroids. *J Am Acad Dermatol* 54: 1–15; quiz 16–18
23 Cornell RC, Stoughton RB (1985) Correlation of the vasoconstriction assay and clinical activity in psoriasis. *Arch Dermatol* 121: 63–67
24 Lebwohl M (2005) A clinician's paradigm in the treatment of psoriasis. *J Am Acad Dermatol* 53: S59–69
25 Thomas KS, Armstrong S, Avery A, Po AL, O'Neill C, Young S, Williams HC (2002) Randomised controlled trial of short bursts of a potent topical corticosteroid *versus* prolonged use of a mild preparation for children with mild or moderate atopic eczema. *BMJ* 324: 768
26 Lebwohl MG, Tan MH, Meador SL, Singer G (2001) Limited application of fluticasone propionate ointment, 0.005% in patients with psoriasis of the face and intertriginous areas. *J Am Acad Dermatol* 44: 77–82
27 Pardasani AG, Feldman SR, Clark AR (2000) Treatment of psoriasis: an algorithm-based approach for primary care physicians. *Am Fam Physician* 61: 725–733, 736
28 Lebwohl M, Peets E, Chen V (1993) Limited application of mometasone furoate on the face and intertriginous areas: analysis of safety and efficacy. *Int J Dermatol* 32: 830–831
29 Korting HC, Kerscher MJ, Schafer-Korting M (1992) Topical glucocorticoids with improved benefit/risk ratio: do they exist? *J Am Acad Dermatol* 27: 87–92
30 Schafer-Korting M, Schmid MH, Korting HC (1996) Topical glucocorticoids with improved risk-benefit ratio. Rationale of a new concept. *Drug Saf* 14: 375–385
31 Huang X, Tanojo H, Lenn J, Deng CH, Krochmal L (2005) A novel foam vehicle for delivery of topical corticosteroids. *J Am Acad Dermatol* 53: S26–38
32 Stein L (2005) Clinical studies of a new vehicle formulation for topical corticosteroids in the treatment of psoriasis. *J Am Acad Dermatol* 53: S39–49
33 Franz TJ, Parsell DA, Myers JA, Hannigan JF (2000) Clobetasol propionate foam 0.05%: a novel vehicle with enhanced delivery. *Int J Dermatol* 39: 535–538
34 Franz TJ, Parsell DA, Halualani RM, Hannigan JF, Kalbach JP, Harkonen WS (1999) Betamethasone valerate foam 0.12%: a novel vehicle with enhanced delivery and efficacy. *Int J Dermatol* 38: 628–632
35 Lebwohl M, Menter A, Koo J, Feldman SR (2004) Combination therapy to treat moderate to severe psoriasis. *J Am Acad Dermatol* 50: 416–430
36 Meola T Jr, Soter NA, Lim HW (1991) Are topical corticosteroids useful adjunctive therapy for the treatment of psoriasis with ultraviolet radiation? A review of the literature. *Arch Dermatol* 127: 1708–1713
37 Schmoll M, Henseler T, Christophers E (1978) Evaluation of PUVA, topical corticosteroids and the combination of both in the treatment of psoriasis. *Br J Dermatol* 99: 693–702
38 Morison WL, Parrish JA, Fitzpatrick TB (1978) Controlled study of PUVA and adjunctive topical therapy in the management of psoriasis. *Br J Dermatol* 98: 125–132
39 Morimoto S, Kumahara Y (1985) A patient with psoriasis cured by 1 alpha-hydroxyvitamin D3. *Med J Osaka Univ* 35: 51–54
40 Smith EL, Walworth NC, Holick MF (1986) Effect of 1 alpha,25-dihydroxyvitamin D3 on the morphologic and biochemical differentiation of cultured human epidermal keratinocytes grown in serum-free conditions. *J Invest Dermatol* 86: 709–714
41 Hosomi J, Hosoi J, Abe E, Suda T, Kuroki T (1983) Regulation of terminal differentiation of cultured mouse epidermal cells by 1 alpha,25-dihydroxyvitamin D3. *Endocrinology* 113: 1950–1957
42 Evans RM (1988) The steroid and thyroid hormone receptor superfamily. *Science* 240: 889–895
43 Binderup L, Bramm E (1988) Effects of a novel vitamin D analogue MC903 on cell proliferation and differentiation *in vitro* and on calcium metabolism *in vivo*. *Biochem Pharmacol* 37: 889–895
44 Lee E, Jeon SH, Yi JY, Jin YJ, Son YS (2001) Calcipotriol inhibits autocrine phosphorylation of EGF receptor in a calcium-dependent manner, a possible mechanism for its inhibition of cell proliferation and stimulation of cell differentiation. *Biochem Biophys Res Commun* 284: 419–425
45 Kragballe K, Wildfang IL (1990) Calcipotriol (MC 903), a novel vitamin D3 analogue stimulates terminal differentiation and inhibits proliferation of cultured human keratinocytes. *Arch Dermatol Res* 282: 164–167
46 Nagpal S, Lu J, Boehm MF (2001) Vitamin D analogs: mechanism of action and therapeutic applications. *Curr Med Chem* 8: 1661–1679
47 Kragballe K, Gjertsen BT, De Hoop D, Karlsmark T, van de Kerkhof PC, Larko O, Nieboer C,

Roed-Petersen J, Strand A, Tikjob G (1991) Double-blind, right/left comparison of calcipotriol and betamethasone valerate in treatment of psoriasis vulgaris. *Lancet* 337: 193–196
48 Cunliffe WJ, Berth-Jones J, Claudy A, Fairiss G, Goldin D, Gratton D, Henderson CA, Holden CA, Maddin WS, Ortonne JP et al. (1992) Comparative study of calcipotriol (MC 903) ointment and betamethasone 17-valerate ointment in patients with psoriasis vulgaris. *J Am Acad Dermatol* 26: 736–743
49 Perez A, Chen TC, Turner A, Raab R, Bhawan J, Poche P, Holick MF (1996) Efficacy and safety of topical calcitriol (1,25-dihydroxyvitamin d3) for the treatment of psoriasis. *Br J Dermatol* 134: 238–246
50 van de Kerkhof PC, Berth-Jones J, Griffiths CE, Harrison PV, Honigsmann H, Marks R, Roelandts R, Schopf E, Trompke C (2002) Long-term efficacy and safety of tacalcitol ointment in patients with chronic plaque psoriasis. *Br J Dermatol* 146: 414–422
51 Mortensen L, Kragballe K, Wegmann E, Schifter S, Risteli J, Charles P (1993) Treatment of psoriasis vulgaris with topical calcipotriol has no short-term effect on calcium or bone metabolism. A randomized, double-blind, placebo-controlled study. *Acta Derm Venereol* 73: 300–304
52 Berth-Jones J, Bourke JF, Iqbal SJ, Hutchinson PE (1993) Urine calcium excretion during treatment of psoriasis with topical calcipotriol. *Br J Dermatol* 129: 411–414
53 Georgiou S, Tsambaos D (1999) Hypercalcaemia and hypercalciuria after topical treatment of psoriasis with excessive amounts of calcipotriol. *Acta Derm Venereol* 79: 86
54 Bourke JF, Berth-Jones J, Iqbal SJ, Hutchinson PE (1993) High-dose topical calcipotriol in the treatment of extensive psoriasis vulgaris. *Br J Dermatol* 129: 74–76
55 Russell S, Young MJ (1994) Hypercalcaemia during treatment of psoriasis with calcipotriol. *Br J Dermatol* 130: 795–796
56 Hardman KA, Heath DA, Nelson HM (1993) Hypercalcaemia associated with calcipotriol (Dovonex) treatment. *BMJ* 306: 896
57 Kawaguchi M, Mitsuhashi Y, Kondo S (2003) Iatrogenic hypercalcemia due to vitamin D3 ointment (1,24(OH)2D3) combined with thiazide diuretics in a case of psoriasis. *J Dermatol* 30: 801–804
58 Tauscher AE, Fleischer AB Jr, Phelps KC, Feldman SR (2002) Psoriasis and pregnancy. *J Cutan Med Surg* 6: 561–570
59 Darley CR, Cunliffe WJ, Green CM, Hutchinson PE, Klaber MR, Downes N (1996) Safety and efficacy of calcipotriol ointment (Dovonex) in treating children with psoriasis vulgaris. *Br J Dermatol* 135: 390–393
60 Oranje AP, Marcoux D, Svensson A, Prendiville J, Krafchik B, Toole J, Rosenthal D, de Waard-van der Spek FB, Molin L, Axelsen M (1997) Topical calcipotriol in childhood psoriasis. *J Am Acad Dermatol* 36: 203–208
61 Kragballe K, Beck HI, Sogaard H (1988) Improvement of psoriasis by a topical vitamin D3 analogue (MC 903) in a double-blind study. *Br J Dermatol* 119: 223–230
62 Kragballe K (1989) Treatment of psoriasis by the topical application of the novel cholecalciferol analogue calcipotriol (MC 903). *Arch Dermatol* 125: 1647–1652
63 Dubertret L, Wallach D, Souteyrand P, Perussel M, Kalis B, Meynadier J, Chevrant-Breton J, Beylot C, Bazex JA, Jurgensen HJ (1992) Efficacy and safety of calcipotriol (MC 903) ointment in psoriasis vulgaris. A randomized, double-blind, right/left comparative, vehicle-controlled study. *J Am Acad Dermatol* 27: 983–988
64 Berardesca E, Vignoli GP, Farinelli N, Vignini M, Distante F, Rabbiosi G (1994) Non-invasive evaluation of topical calcipotriol *versus* clobetasol in the treatment of psoriasis. *Acta Derm Venereol* 74: 302–304
65 Bruce S, Epinette WW, Funicella T, Ison A, Jones EL, Loss R Jr, McPhee ME, Whitmore C (1994) Comparative study of calcipotriene (MC 903) ointment and fluocinonide ointment in the treatment of psoriasis. *J Am Acad Dermatol* 31: 755–759
66 Camarasa JM, Ortonne JP, Dubertret L (2003) Calcitriol shows greater persistence of treatment effect than betamethasone dipropionate in topical psoriasis therapy. *J Dermatolog Treat* 14: 8–13
67 Wall AR, Poyner TF, Menday AP (1998) A comparison of treatment with dithranol and calcipotriol on the clinical severity and quality of life in patients with psoriasis. *Br J Dermatol* 139: 1005–1011
68 Thaci D, Daiber W, Boehncke WH, Kaufmann R (2001) Calcipotriol solution for the treatment of scalp psoriasis: evaluation of efficacy, safety and acceptance in 3'396 patients. *Dermatology* 203: 153–156
69 Ortonne JP, Humbert P, Nicolas JF, Tsankov N, Tonev SD, Janin A, Czernielewski J, Lahfa M,

Dubertret L (2003) Intra-individual comparison of the cutaneous safety and efficacy of calcitriol 3 microg g(−1) ointment and calcipotriol 50 microg g(−1) ointment on chronic plaque psoriasis localized in facial, hairline, retroauricular or flexural areas. *Br J Dermatol* 148: 326–333
70 Takahashi H, Ibe M, Kinouchi M, Ishida-Yamamoto A, Hashimoto Y, Iizuka H (2003) Similarly potent action of 1,25-dihydroxyvitamin D3 and its analogues, tacalcitol, calcipotriol, and maxacalcitol on normal human keratinocyte proliferation and differentiation. *J Dermatol Sci* 31: 21–28
71 Van de Kerkhof PC, Werfel T, Haustein UF, Luger T, Czarnetzki BM, Niemann R, Planitz-Stenzel V (1996) Tacalcitol ointment in the treatment of psoriasis vulgaris: a multicentre, placebo-controlled, double-blind study on efficacy and safety. *Br J Dermatol* 135: 758–765
72 Veien NK, Bjerke JR, Rossmann-Ringdahl I, Jakobsen HB (1997) Once daily treatment of psoriasis with tacalcitol compared with twice daily treatment with calcipotriol. A double-blind trial. *Br J Dermatol* 137: 581–586
73 Barker JN, Ashton RE, Marks R, Harris RI, Berth-Jones J (1999) Topical maxacalcitol for the treatment of psoriasis vulgaris: a placebo-controlled, double-blind, dose-finding study with active comparator. *Br J Dermatol* 141: 274–278
74 Durakovic C, Ray S, Holick MF (2004) Topical paricalcitol (19-nor-1 alpha,25-dihydroxyvitamin D2) is a novel, safe and effective treatment for plaque psoriasis: a pilot study. *Br J Dermatol* 151: 190–195
75 Lebwohl M, Siskin SB, Epinette W, Breneman D, Funicella T, Kalb R, Moore J (1996) A multicenter trial of calcipotriene ointment and halobetasol ointment compared with either agent alone for the treatment of psoriasis. *J Am Acad Dermatol* 35: 268–269
76 Lebwohl M, Yoles A, Lombardi K, Lou W (1998) Calcipotriene ointment and halobetasol ointment in the long-term treatment of psoriasis: effects on the duration of improvement. *J Am Acad Dermatol* 39: 447–450
77 Douglas WS, Poulin Y, Decroix J, Ortonne JP, Mrowietz U, Gulliver W, Krogstad AL, Larsen FG, Iglesias L, Buckley C et al. (2002) A new calcipotriol/betamethasone formulation with rapid onset of action was superior to monotherapy with betamethasone dipropionate or calcipotriol in psoriasis vulgaris. *Acta Derm Venereol* 82: 131–135
78 Papp KA, Guenther L, Boyden B, Larsen FG, Harvima RJ, Guilhou JJ, Kaufmann R, Rogers S, van de Kerkhof PC, Hanssen LI et al. (2003) Early onset of action and efficacy of a combination of calcipotriene and betamethasone dipropionate in the treatment of psoriasis. *J Am Acad Dermatol* 48: 48–54
79 Guenther L, Van de Kerkhof PC, Snellman E, Kragballe K, Chu AC, Tegner E, Garcia-Diez A, Springborg J (2002) Efficacy and safety of a new combination of calcipotriol and betamethasone dipropionate (once or twice daily) compared to calcipotriol (twice daily) in the treatment of psoriasis vulgaris: a randomized, double-blind, vehicle-controlled clinical trial. *Br J Dermatol* 147: 316–323
80 Ortonne JP, Kaufmann R, Lecha M, Goodfield M (2004) Efficacy of treatment with calcipotriol/betamethasone dipropionate followed by calcipotriol alone compared with tacalcitol for the treatment of psoriasis vulgaris: a randomised, double-blind trial. *Dermatology* 209: 308–313
81 Kragballe K, Noerrelund KL, Lui H, Ortonne JP, Wozel G, Uurasmaa T, Fleming C, Estebaranz JL, Hanssen LI, Persson LM (2004) Efficacy of once-daily treatment regimens with calcipotriol/betamethasone dipropionate ointment and calcipotriol ointment in psoriasis vulgaris. *Br J Dermatol* 150: 1167–1173
82 Kragballe K, Austad J, Barnes L, Bibby A, de la Brassinne M, Cambazard F, Fleming C, Heikkila H, Jolliffe D, Peyri J et al. (2006) A 52-week randomized safety study of a calcipotriol/betamethasone dipropionate two-compound product (Dovobet/Daivobet/Taclonex) in the treatment of psoriasis vulgaris. *Br J Dermatol* 154: 1155–1160
83 Kragballe K, Austad J, Barnes L, Bibby A, de la Brassinne M, Cambazard F, Fleming C, Heikkila H, Williams Z, Peyri Rey J et al. (2006) Efficacy results of a 52-week, randomised, double-blind, safety study of a calcipotriol/betamethasone dipropionate two-compound product (Daivobet/Dovobet/Taclonex) in the treatment of psoriasis vulgaris. *Dermatology* 213: 319–326
84 White S, Vender R, Thaci D, Haverkamp C, Naeyaert JM, Foster R, Martinez Escribano JA, Cambazard F, Bibby A (2006) Use of calcipotriene cream (Dovonex cream) following acute treatment of psoriasis vulgaris with the calcipotriene/betamethasone dipropionate two-compound product (Taclonex): a randomized, parallel-group clinical trial. *Am J Clin Dermatol* 7: 177–184
85 Kragballe K, van de Kerkhof PC (2006) Consistency of data in six phase III clinical studies of a two-compound product containing calcipotriol and betamethasone dipropionate ointment for the

treatment of psoriasis. *J Eur Acad Dermatol Venereol* 20: 39–44
86 Blum RR, Stern D, Lebwohl M, Bandow G, Koo J, Cheplo K (2004) A multi-center study of calcipotriene ointment, 0.005% and clobetasol propionate foam, 0.05% in the sequential treatment of localized plaque-type psoriasis. *Summer Meeting of the American Academy of Dermatology*, New York, NY
87 Koo J, Blum RR, Lebwohl M (2006) A randomized, multicenter study of calcipotriene ointment and clobetasol propionate foam in the sequential treatment of localized plaque-type psoriasis: short- and long-term outcomes. *J Am Acad Dermatol* 55: 637–641
88 Bowman PH, Maloney JE, Koo JY (2002) Combination of calcipotriene (Dovonex) ointment and tazarotene (Tazorac) gel *versus* clobetasol ointment in the treatment of plaque psoriasis: a pilot study. *J Am Acad Dermatol* 46: 907–913
89 Patel B, Siskin S, Krazmien R, Lebwohl M (1998) Compatibility of calcipotriene with other topical medications. *J Am Acad Dermatol* 38: 1010–1011
90 Ashcroft DM, Li Wan Po A, Williams HC, Griffiths CE (2000) Combination regimens of topical calcipotriene in chronic plaque psoriasis: systematic review of efficacy and tolerability. *Arch Dermatol* 136: 1536–1543
91 Hecker D, Lebwohl M (1997) Topical calcipotriene in combination with UVB phototherapy for psoriasis. *Int J Dermatol* 36: 302–303
92 Molin L (1999) Topical calcipotriol combined with phototherapy for psoriasis. The results of two randomized trials and a review of the literature. Calcipotriol-UVB Study Group. *Dermatology* 198: 375–381
93 Kragballe K (1990) Combination of topical calcipotriol (MC 903) and UVB radiation for psoriasis vulgaris. *Dermatologica* 181: 211–214
94 Ramsay CA, Schwartz BE, Lowson D, Papp K, Bolduc A, Gilbert M (2000) Calcipotriol cream combined with twice weekly broad-band UVB phototherapy: a safe, effective and UVB-sparing antipsoriatric combination treatment. The Canadian Calcipotriol and UVB Study Group. *Dermatology* 200: 17–24
95 Brands S, Brakman M, Bos JD, de Rie MA (1999) No additional effect of calcipotriol ointment on low-dose narrow-band UVB phototherapy in psoriasis. *J Am Acad Dermatol* 41: 991–995
96 Frappaz A TJ (1993) Calcipotriol in combination with PUVA: a randomized double placebo study in severe psoriasis. *Eur J Dermatol* 3: 351–354
97 Lebwohl M, Hecker D, Martinez J, Sapadin A, Patel B (1997) Interactions between calcipotriene and ultraviolet light. *J Am Acad Dermatol* 37: 93–95
98 van de Kerkhof PC, Cambazard F, Hutchinson PE, Haneke E, Wong E, Souteyrand P, Damstra RJ, Combemale P, Neumann MH, Chalmers RJ et al. (1998) The effect of addition of calcipotriol ointment (50 micrograms/g) to acitretin therapy in psoriasis. *Br J Dermatol* 138: 84–89
99 de Jong EM, Mork NJ, Seijger MM, De La Brassine M, Lauharanta J, Jansen CT, Guilhou JJ, Guillot B, Ostrojic A, Souteyrand P et al. (2003) The combination of calcipotriol and methotrexate compared with methotrexate and vehicle in psoriasis: results of a multicentre placebo-controlled randomized trial. *Br J Dermatol* 148: 318–325
100 Grossman RM, Thivolet J, Claudy A, Souteyrand P, Guilhou JJ, Thomas P, Amblard P, Belaich S, de Belilovsky C, de la Brassinne M et al. (1994) A novel therapeutic approach to psoriasis with combination calcipotriol ointment and very low-dose cyclosporine: results of a multicenter placebo-controlled study. *J Am Acad Dermatol* 31: 68–74

Topical therapy II: retinoids, immunomodulators, and others

Paru R. Chaudhari, Dana K. Stern and Mark G. Lebwohl

Mount Sinai School of Medicine Department of Dermatology, 5 E 98th St 5th Floor, New York, NY 10029, USA

Introduction

Use of topical therapy for mild and moderate psoriasis continues to be a mainstay of treatment. The previous chapter introduced topical corticosteroids and vitamin D analogs as the most common therapies for psoriasis (see Tab. 1). Here the newly available topical retinoids and immunomodulators, along with the traditional therapies of tars, anthralin, and salicylic acid, will be discussed in detail.

Table 1. Topical psoriasis treatments

Anthralin
Corticosteroids
Salicylic acid
Tar
Tazarotene
Topical immunomodulators
Vitamin D analogs

Topical retinoids

Mechanism of action

Topical retinoids were first introduced as treatment for psoriasis in 1997 [1]. Tazarotene, the only approved topical retinoid available for the treatment of psoriasis, acts on psoriatic lesions after conversion by esterases in the skin to the active form, tazarotenic acid [2]. The retinoid selectively binds to β and γ-retinoic acid receptors (RAR) on the cell membrane of keratinocytes and is then transported to the nucleus, altering transcription of genes in keratinocytes [2, 3]. Specifically, TIG (tazarotene-induced genes) 1, 2 and 3, have been shown to reduce keratinocyte proliferation when stimulated by topical tazarotene [4–6]. TIG3 has been further identified as a tumor suppressor and growth regulator gene. Tazarotene also suppresses the migration inhibitory factor-related protein 8 (MRP8), a marker for inflammation normally seen at high levels in psoriasis [7]. Thus, topical retinoids can reduce keratinocyte proliferation, lessen inflammation and normalize keratinocyte differentiation, all factors that contribute to psoriatic lesions.

Adverse effects

Pruritus, burning, erythema and irritant contact dermatitis are the most common adverse events associated with topical tazarotene application, occurring in up to 30% of patients [7]. Side effects are generally more pronounced with the 0.1% tazarotene concentration than with the 0.05% concentration [8, 9].

Due to the conversion of tazarotene into tazarotenic acid by esterases in the skin, the topical retinoid is minimally absorbed into the bloodstream. After 12 weeks of tazarotene therapy in several Phase III clinical studies, less than 3% of patients showed detectable levels of retinoid in the blood and no systemic adverse events were reported [8–10]. However, as with most topical therapies for psoriasis, tazarotene should not be used on greater than 20% of the body surface area due to an increase in systemic absorption.

Use of topical retinoids in pregnancy and in pediatric populations

Tazarotene is contraindicated in pregnancy, Category X (see Tab. 2), because of the theoretical risk of teratogenicity [11]. Therefore, women of child-bear-

Table 2. Categories for drug use during pregnancy

Category A	Adequate and well-controlled studies have failed to demonstrate a risk to the fetus in the first trimester of pregnancy (and there is no evidence of risk in later trimesters).
Category B	Animal reproduction studies have failed to demonstrate a risk to the fetus and there are no adequate and well-controlled studies in pregnant women OR Animal studies have shown an adverse effect, but adequate and well-controlled studies in pregnant women have failed to demonstrate a risk to the fetus in any trimester.
Category C	Animal reproduction studies have shown an adverse effect on the fetus and there are no adequate and well-controlled studies in humans, but potential benefits may warrant use of the drug in pregnant women despite potential risks.
Category D	There is positive evidence of human fetal risk based on adverse reaction data from investigational or marketing experience or studies in humans, but potential benefits may warrant use of the drug in pregnant women despite potential risks.
Category X	Studies in animals or humans have demonstrated fetal abnormalities and/or there is positive evidence of human fetal risk based on adverse reaction data from investigational or marketing experience, and the risks involved in use of the drug in pregnant women clearly outweigh potential benefits.

Reprinted from http://www.fda.gov/fdac/features/2001/301_preg.html#categories

ing age should be warned about the risks of becoming pregnant during topical retinoid therapy and be counseled about birth control. Children tolerate topical retinoids well, demonstrating side effects similar in type and severity to those in adults. Topical retinoids are therefore considered safe and efficacious in the pediatric population, although no specific trials have been conducted with children or adolescents, and it remains an off-label use of the medication.

Therapeutic response

Non-steroidal therapies for psoriasis such as tazarotene are highly attractive due to the undesirable side effects of corticosteroid therapy. Topical tazarotene has been found effective for the treatment of psoriasis in multiple clinical trials and is available as a gel or cream in 0.05% and 0.1% concentrations. In a double-blind, randomized, vehicle-controlled trial, once-a-day tazarotene gel significantly reduced psoriatic plaque elevation, scaling and to a lesser degree erythema after 12 weeks of therapy [9]. Target lesions showed 70% clearance rates with the 0.1% gel and 59% with the 0.05% gel. In two multicenter, double-blind, randomized, vehicle-controlled trials, tazarotene cream also improved psoriatic lesions [8]. After 12 weeks of treatment, the 0.1% cream was found more effective but caused greater skin irritation than the 0.05% cream. In addition, both gel and cream vehicles maintained clearance in approximately 40–50% of target lesions 12 weeks post-treatment [8, 9].

Tazarotene has been demonstrated to be an effective maintenance therapy for psoriasis. A randomized, multicenter, investigator-masked, parallel group study that compared twice-daily fluocinonide 0.05% ointment to once-daily tazarotene 0.1% gel demonstrated that relapse rates for tazarotene gel were 18% as opposed to 55% for fluocinonide in the 12 weeks post-treatment [12]. In this study, the potent corticosteroid was superior at treating erythema but not target lesions. Tazarotene has also been compared to vitamin D analogs. Treatment with once-daily tazarotene 0.1% gel plus petrolatum for 12 weeks was as effective as twice-daily calcipotriol 0.005% ointment during an investigator-blind, bilateral comparison trial for plaque psoriasis [13]. Tazarotene sustained its therapeutic effect four weeks post-treatment, providing further evidence for its use as a maintenance therapy. In general, tazarotene is indicated for stable plaque psoriasis but is usually prescribed in combination with other psoriasis therapy.

Bexarotene gel, a synthetic topical retinoid traditionally used to treat cutaneous T cell lymphoma, is being studied as a potential topical treatment for psoriasis. In a recent double-blind, randomized, vehicle-controlled trial, bexarotene 1% gel combined with narrowband ultraviolet B (NBUVB) was significantly more effective at treating psoriasis than NBUVB alone [14]. Further clinical studies, however, are necessary to determine the extent of its efficacy as a monotherapy.

Topical retinoids as combination therapy

Combinations of tazarotene with other topical therapies, UV light and systemic agents have been studied for the treatment of psoriasis. For example, tazarotene coupled with topical corticosteroids clears psoriatic lesions more effectively than does either agent alone [15–20]. The combination significantly reduces adverse effects as well, and thus tazarotene is typically prescribed as part of a combined regimen. In an investigator-masked, multicenter trial, tazarotene coupled with mid- and high-potency corticosteroids for 12 weeks significantly reduced psoriatic scaling and side effects such as skin irritation. Benefits persisted in the 4 weeks post-treatment [15]. In addition, Koo et al., reported that once-daily mometasone furoate 0.1% combined with once-daily tazarotene 0.1% gel for 12 weeks was more effective than either tazarotene or mometasone furoate alone, suggesting a synergistic effect [18]. Alternate day therapy with topical corticosteroids and tazarotene is another effective treatment regimen for psoriasis. In a multicenter, double-blind, parallel group study, alternate day therapy with tazarotene 0.1% gel and clobetasol ointment for 12 weeks reduced scaling and erythema while decreasing side effects by 50% [16]. Topical retinoids have also been combined with vitamin D analogs. A pilot study with 15 patients concluded that twice-daily calcipotriol ointment plus once-daily tazarotene gel was equivalent to twice-daily clobetasol ointment in reducing psoriatic scaling, plaque elevation, and severity of lesions after 2 weeks of treatment [21]. This study demonstrated the stability of vitamin D analogs when combined with tazarotene. The vitamin D/tazarotene combination may eventually prove to be an effective alternative to steroid-based regimens.

Tazarotene combined with either ultraviolet-B (UVB) or psoralen plus ultraviolet-A (PUVA) is an effective treatment regimen for psoriasis [22, 23]. After 10 weeks of therapy in an investigator-blinded, bilateral comparison trial, 80% of subjects treated with the UVB/tazarotene combination experienced improvement of their psoriasis compared to only 50% of subjects exposed to UVB alone [24]. The cumulative UVB dose necessary to treat psoriasis was significantly lower with the combination therapy. In addition, NBUVB plus tazarotene is more effective at clearing psoriasis than NBUVB alone. In a 10 patient, right-left comparison trial, the combination significantly improved psoriatic lesions after 4 weeks of treatment [25]. While the actions of tazarotene and UVB appear to be synergistic, the application of tazarotene leads to thinning of protective layers in the epidermis necessitating a one-third reduction of the normal UVB dose to prevent phototoxicity [26]. Tazarotene and PUVA therapy has also been successfully combined for the treatment of psoriasis. Significant improvement was noted in 12 patients receiving 4 weeks of PUVA/tazarotene compared to PUVA/vehicle during a right-to-left comparison trial [27]. Tanew et al. also concluded that PUVA plus tazarotene is more effective than PUVA alone against plaque-type psoriasis [28]. This combination lowered the cumulative dose of UVA necessary to achieve clearance, decreasing the long-term risks of skin malignancy due to PUVA therapy. As with UVB, lower UVA doses are required when coupled with tazarotene [26].

Topical immunomodulators

Mechanism of action

Tacrolimus (FK-506) and pimecrolimus (SDZ ASM 981) are two topical calcium-dependent phosphatase (calcineurin) inhibitors that can downregulate antigen-specific T cell reactivity [29]. They bind to macrophilin-12 (FKBP-12), blocking calcium signal transduction in T lymphocytes by impeding nuclear factor of activated T cells (NF-AT) [30]. Topical immunomodulators inhibit transcription of inflammatory cytokines, including interleukin (IL)-2, IL-3, IL-4, IL-5, interferon (IFN)-γ and tumor necrosis factor (TNF)-α, which normally contribute to psoriatic lesions. Topical immunomodulators can also inhibit mast cell degranulation, preventing the release of histamine, cytokines and other inflammatory factors that contribute to the pathogenesis of psoriasis [31–33].

Adverse effects

Local side effects of topical immunomodulators include mild to moderate skin irritation accompanied by burning and pruritus at the site of application [34]. The use of tacrolimus and pimecrolimus is approved by the Food and Drug Administration (FDA) for the treatment of atopic dermatitis (AD) only; therefore, most studies concerning the safety of topical immunomodulators focus on patients with AD. Topical adverse effects of the immunomodulators may actually occur less frequently on the thick plaques of psoriasis [29]. In head-to-head randomized trials comparing tacrolimus to pimecrolimus, one study reported an equal rate of burning between the two drugs while another concluded that pimecrolimus had a better local side effect profile. Tacrolimus was more effective for atopic dermatitis in the latter study [35, 36].

Due to the minimal systemic absorption of topical immunomodulators, systemic toxicity is less of a concern than it is with oral administration [37]. Occasionally, patients using topical immunomodulators experience flu-like symptoms, headaches, folliculitis and increased flushing after alcohol use [34]. Serious adverse effects in patients with atopic dermatitis have included staphylococcal superinfection, eczema herpeticum, varicella and cellulitis; it is unclear whether these events occurred as a result of the AD itself or as a result of medication usage [38]. High systemic absorption of topical immunomodulators has been reported in patients with severe skin disruption; therefore, treatments are not recommended in patients with significant barrier interruption or other systemic illnesses such as mononucleosis [39].

Recently, the FDA has raised concern about the safety of topical immunomodulators. As a result, they have issued a black-box warning regarding the use of both tacrolimus and pimecrolimus [40]. This concern is based on evidence of malignancy after long-term use of oral immunosuppressants and reported cases of malignancies possibly related to topical immunomodulators. Topical immunomodulators have been shown *in vitro* to inhibit DNA repair in keratinocytes, potentially leading to an increased risk of malignancy [41, 42]. Oral pimecrolimus has also been shown to cause lymphoma in animals, but with serum concentrations of the drug over 30 times those normally seen in humans [43, 44]. Topical immunomodulators were also shown to increase the risk of lymphoma in mice, but at doses much greater than those used in humans [41, 45]. As a result, new FDA recommendations state that topical immunomodulators should not be used as long-term treatment, over large surface areas, or in children under the age of two. However, the FDA also mentions that no casual relationship has been established between the use of topical immunomodulators and the reported cases of malignancy [46].

Clinical evidence up to this point does not show an enhanced risk of cancer after use of either topical tacrolimus or pimecrolimus; malignancy rates in patients treated with topical immunomodulators are equal to what is expected in the normal population [47]. Many medical professional societies also support the use of pimecrolimus and tacrolimus. Further investigations regarding the safety of topical immunomodulators are underway [41, 46]. Because topical immunomodulator therapy is not an approved treatment for psoriasis, risks and benefits of the medications should be carefully considered and discussed with patients [48].

Use of topical immunomodulators in pregnancy and in pediatric populations

Both topical tacrolimus and pimecrolimus have been labeled Category C (see Tab. 2), but are generally not considered teratogenic due to their low systemic absorption [11]. Oral tacrolimus has been reported to cause preterm births and teratogenic events, and thus close monitoring of pregnant patients is advised when using topical immunomodulator therapy [49]. In addition, pregnant patients should be educated about the use of topical immunomodulator therapy for psoriasis because long-term consequences are unknown and it remains an off-label use of the medication.

Treatment with topical immunomodulators has been studied in younger patients with atopic dermatitis, but only minimal evidence exists regarding psoriasis in the same age range. The safety and tolerability of pimecrolimus 1% cream was described in over 1'000 infants with AD [50]. A recent retrospective study described improvement in 12 out of 13 patients with pediatric inverse psoriasis using tacrolimus 0.1% ointment daily with minimal reported side effects [51]. Because of the large surface-to-volume ratio of infants and young children, systemic absorption of topical immunomodulators is enhanced and they should be carefully monitored. There is uncertainty regarding long-term side effects in pediatric patients with AD, and no long-term studies have been done on young patients with psoriasis.

Therapeutic effect

Despite the efficacy for the treatment of atopic dermatitis, once-daily topical tacrolimus 0.3% ointment was found to be ineffective for the treatment of non-intertriginous psoriatic plaques between 40 cm^2 and 200 cm^2 in size [52]. This lack of efficacy was attributed to the inability of tacrolimus to penetrate thick, psoriatic plaques due to its large molecular size. When placed under occlusion on descaled microplaques, however, topical tacrolimus was found to be an effective treatment for psoriasis [53].

Plaque psoriasis of the face and intertriginous areas tends to be thin and thus more responsive to tacrolimus therapy. Because topical immunomodulators do not cause skin atrophy or changes in collagen synthesis, they are highly attractive therapies for inverse psoriasis [54, 55]. Lebwohl et al. demonstrated an 81% clearance rate in 21 patients with inverse psoriasis after treatment with twice-daily tacrolimus 0.1% ointment for 8 weeks [56]. Twice-daily therapy with tacrolimus 0.1% ointment for 4 weeks was demonstrated to be effective for facial psoriasis [57, 58]. In a randomized, double-blind 8 week trial, the efficacy of topical tacrolimus 0.1% ointment for the treatment of inverse psoriasis was corroborated, demonstrating improvement in erythema, desquamation induration, and overall severity [59]. Topical tacrolimus may be beneficial in pustular psoriasis as well [60].

Newer vehicles of topical tacrolimus, a 0.3% gel and 0.5% cream, have been developed in order to more effectively penetrate thick psoriatic plaques. In a recent randomized, open-label, observer-blind study, tacrolimus 0.3% gel was found to be equivalent to 0.005% calcipotriol ointment for the treatment of mild-to-moderate plaque psoriasis. However, lesions that received the vitamin D analog had a faster rate improvement [61]. In this trial, the tacrolimus 0.5% cream was less effective than both tacrolimus 0.3% gel and the calcipotriol 0.005% ointment. Further studies are needed to evaluate the newer vehicles.

Pimecrolimus 1% is effective when applied to microplaques under occlusion [62]. Because topical pimecrolimus does not cause skin atrophy, its use on sensitive areas of the body is also appropriate [55]. Inverse psoriasis significantly improved with twice-daily 1% pimecrolimus cream for 8 weeks in a double-blind, randomized, vehicle-controlled study with 57 patients [63]. Pimecrolimus may improve psoriatic plaques without occlusion as well. In a double-blind, randomized study, twice-daily pimecrolimus 1% ointment (with 10% urea) was found to be more effective than placebo at treating psoriatic plaques, but less effective than either topical corticosteroids or vitamin D analogs [64]. Sirolimus, a newly created topical immunomodulator, has recently been investigated as a possible treatment for psoriasis with promising initial study results [65].

Topical immunomodulators as combination therapy

In a recent right-left comparison trial of 24 patients, the combination of twice-daily salicylic acid 6% gel and once-daily tacrolimus 0.1% ointment resulted in significant improvement of psoriatic plaques in comparison to salicylic acid alone [66]. Although the exact mechanism is unknown, it is hypothesized that salicylic acid may improve the absorption of topical immunomodulators.

Other topical treatments

Tars

Topical tars have been used for the treatment of cutaneous disorders, including psoriasis, for over 100 years [67]. The Goeckerman regimen, first reported in 1925, successfully combined coal tar with UV radiation to treat psoriatic lesions [68]. Decades later, the mechanism of action of coal tar is still not completely clear. It has been shown to lessen mitotic index labeling and suppress DNA synthesis in keratinocytes, an effect enhanced by exposure to UV radiation [69]. The original Goeckerman regimen included tar placement on psoriatic patches with a gradual increase in exposure to UV radiation, performed on an inpatient basis. Later, the modified ambulatory Goeckerman regimen (MAGR) included coal tar at bedtime with exposure to UV the following morning [70]. Variations of the Goeckerman regimen have been used for the last 80 years and have been extremely effective treatment strategies [71]. The success of coal tar has been demonstrated on chronic plaque and scalp psoriasis [26]. Most chronic plaques generally improve after 1 month and patients remain in remission for longer than with other psoriatic topical therapies [72]. In a recent double-blinded, randomized study, the newly developed coal tar 1% lotion was found to be superior to the more common 5% preparation at treating chronic plaque-type psoriasis [73]. The use of tar, however, has waned due to its poor side effect profile and superior efficacy of alternative topical therapies [26]. Adverse effects of coal tar include odor, staining, irritant contact dermatitis, erythema, stinging, folliculitis and formation of keratoacanthomas [74]. Coal tar was as effective as calcipotriol after 12 weeks of therapy in a prospective study; however, the vitamin D analog was better tolerated and had a faster onset of action [75]. Despite the availability of newer, more tolerable topical agents, coal tar remains a first-line agent in much of the world because of its availability and low cost [76]. In the US the Goeckerman regimen is now largely limited to treatment-resistant situations, and can be synergistically coupled with other therapies such as acitretin and narrowband UVB [71].

Anthralin

Anthralin, also known as dithranol, is derived from the Arroba tree and has been used for the treatment of psoriasis for many decades [77]. Because of its chemical instability, anthralin must be formulated in a precise and consistent manner. It is available as 0.1% and 1.0% concentrations in lotion, ointment or paste vehicles. Although the exact mechanism of action is unclear, anthralin is able to reduce keratinocyte proliferation, prevent T cell activation and restore cell differentiation, probably through mitochondrial dysfunction [78]. In addition, the therapy forms free radicals, which may also contribute to its effect against psoriasis [79]. The Ingram technique was first described in 1953, which included daily tar baths and UVB therapy followed by application of anthralin paste to psoriatic lesions. After additional application of talcum powder, the treatment was left on lesions for 24 h and then washed off [80, 81]. Although the regimen is effective at treating psoriasis, anthralin use is limited due to its side effects, which include skin irritation and staining of skin as well as neighboring objects [26, 80, 82]. As a result, regimens have been developed to counteract the unpleasant side effects of the therapy. In a 36 subject inpatient study, short-contact anthralin was found equivalent to normal anthralin on chronic-plaque type psoriasis, but with lower rates of skin irritation and staining [83, 84]. Micanol, which contains 1% anthralin, becomes activated only at skin temperature, reducing staining on neighboring objects while maintaining efficacy [85]. In addition, application of 10% trienthanolamine, a nonsteroidal chemical, lessens the staining created by dithranal by neutralizing any anthralin residue remaining on the skin [86]. Although the combination of anthralin and tar was once popular, evidence now suggests that application of coal tar may inactivate anthralin [87, 88].

Salicylic acid

Salicylic acid, a topical keratolytic, has been used to treat psoriasis for many years. The keratolytic effects of salicylic acid may occur by reducing intercellular bonding in the epidermal layer as well as reducing the pH of the stratum corneum, causing softening of psoriatic lesions [89–91]. Salicylic acid is generally combined with other topical therapies for psoriasis. When topical corticosteroids and salicylic acid are used together, the efficacy of topical corticosteroids is significantly improved due to enhanced skin absorption [92]. This has led to a combined product containing betamethasone dipropionate and salicylic acid, Diprosalic® and Nerisalic®, both of which are available outside of the US [93]. In a multicenter, double-blind, randomized, parallel-group study, twice-daily mometasone furoate 0.1% ointment/salicylic acid 5% ointment for 3 weeks was significantly more effective at treating scaly psoriatic plaques than mometasone furoate alone [94]. Although the combined treatment enhances the therapeutic response, the potential for higher systemic absorptions must be considered. Serum levels of salicylates should be closely monitored in patients on the dual therapy. Tacrolimus and coal tar have also been successfully combined with salicylic acid for the treatment of psoriasis, but calcipotriol loses its efficacy when added to 6% salicylic acid ointment [66, 95]. In addition, salicylic acid blocks UV light and should only be applied after phototherapy [89].

Although systemic absorption is rare, salicylate toxicity has been reported with the use of topical formulations [89]. Toxicity results in changes to the central nervous system including altered mental status, nausea and vomiting, tinnitus and eventually coma [96]. Therefore, application over large portions of the body (>20%), use in patients with renal or hepatic impairment and simultaneous use of other salicylate drugs is not recommended. Because of the greater risk of systemic absorption and toxicity, salicylic should be avoided in children.

References

1 Chandraratna RA (1996) Tazarotene – first of a new generation of receptor-selective retinoids. *Br J Dermatol* 135 Suppl 49: 18–25

2 Duvic M, Nagpal S, Asano AT, Chandraratna RA (1997) Molecular mechanisms of tazarotene action in psoriasis. *J Am Acad Dermatol* 37: S18–24

3 Nagpal S, Athanikar J, Chandraratna RA (1995) Separation of transactivation and AP1 antagonism functions of retinoic acid receptor alpha. *J Biol Chem* 270: 923–927

4 Nagpal S, Patel S, Asano AT, Johnson AT, Duvic M, Chandraratna RA (1996) Tazarotene-induced gene 1 (TIG1), a novel retinoic acid receptor-responsive gene in skin. *J Invest Dermatol* 106: 269–274

5 Nagpal S, Patel S, Jacobe H, DiSepio D, Ghosn C, Malhotra M, Teng M, Duvic M, Chandraratna RA (1997) Tazarotene-induced gene 2 (TIG2), a novel retinoid-responsive gene in skin. *J Invest Dermatol* 109: 91–95

6 DiSepio D, Ghosn C, Eckert RL, Deucher A, Robinson N, Duvic M, Chandraratna RA, Nagpal S (1998) Identification and characterization of a retinoid-induced class II tumor suppressor/growth regulatory gene. *Proc Natl Acad Sci USA* 95: 14811–14815

7 Foster RH, Brogden RN, Benfield P (1998) Tazarotene. *Drugs* 55: 705–711; discussion 712

8 Weinstein GD, Koo JY, Krueger GG, Lebwohl MG, Lowe NJ, Menter MA, Lew-Kaya DA, Sefton J, Gibson JR, Walker PS (2003) Tazarotene cream in the treatment of psoriasis: Two multicenter, double-blind, randomized, vehicle-controlled studies of the safety and efficacy of tazarotene creams 0.05% and 0.1% applied once daily for 12 weeks. *J Am Acad Dermatol* 48: 760–767

9 Weinstein GD, Krueger GG, Lowe NJ, Duvic M, Friedman DJ, Jegasothy BV, Jorizzo JL, Shmunes E, Tschen EH, Lew-Kaya DA et al. (1997) Tazarotene gel, a new retinoid, for topical therapy of psoriasis: vehicle-controlled study of safety, efficacy, and duration of therapeutic effect. *J Am Acad Dermatol* 37: 85–92

10 Tang-Liu DD, Matsumoto RM, Usansky JI (1999) Clinical pharmacokinetics and drug metabolism of tazarotene: a novel topical treatment for acne and psoriasis. *Clin Pharmacokinet* 37: 273–287

11 Tauscher AE, Fleischer AB Jr, Phelps KC, Feldman SR (2002) Psoriasis and pregnancy. *J Cutan Med Surg* 6: 561–570

12 Lebwohl M, Ast E, Callen JP, Cullen SI, Hong SR, Kulp-Shorten CL, Lowe NJ, Phillips TJ, Rosen T, Wolf DI et al. (1998) Once-daily tazarotene gel *versus* twice-daily fluocinonide cream in the treatment of plaque psoriasis. *J Am Acad Dermatol* 38: 705–711

13 Tzung TY, Wu JC, Hsu NJ, Chen YH, Ger LP (2005) Comparison of tazarotene 0.1% gel plus petrolatum once daily *versus* calcipotriol 0.005% ointment twice daily in the treatment of plaque psoriasis. *Acta Derm Venereol* 85: 236–239

14 Magliocco MA, Pandya K, Dombrovskiy V, Christiansen L, Wong Y, Gottlieb AB (2006) A ran-

domized, double-blind, vehicle-controlled, bilateral comparison trial of bexarotene gel 1% *versus* vehicle gel in combination with narrowband UVB phototherapy for moderate to severe psoriasis vulgaris. *J Am Acad Dermatol* 54: 115–118
15 Lebwohl MG, Breneman DL, Goffe BS, Grossman JR, Ling MR, Milbauer J, Pincus SH, Sibbald RG, Swinyer LJ, Weinstein GD et al. (1998) Tazarotene 0.1% gel plus corticosteroid cream in the treatment of plaque psoriasis. *J Am Acad Dermatol* 39: 590–596
16 Gollnick H, Menter A (1999) Combination therapy with tazarotene plus a topical corticosteroid for the treatment of plaque psoriasis. *Br J Dermatol* 140 Suppl 54: 18–23
17 Guenther LC, Poulin YP, Pariser DM (2000) A comparison of tazarotene 0.1% gel once daily plus mometasone furoate 0.1% cream once daily *versus* calcipotriene 0.005% ointment twice daily in the treatment of plaque psoriasis. *Clin Ther* 22: 1225–1238
18 Koo JY, Martin D (2001) Investigator-masked comparison of tazarotene gel q.d. plus mometasone furoate cream q.d. *versus* mometasone furoate cream b.i.d. in the treatment of plaque psoriasis. *Int J Dermatol* 40: 210–212
19 Green L, Sadoff W (2002) A clinical evaluation of tazarotene 0.1% gel, with and without a high- or mid-high-potency corticosteroid, in patients with stable plaque psoriasis. *J Cutan Med Surg* 6: 95–102
20 Dhawan SS, Blyumin ML, Pearce DJ, Feldman SR (2005) Tazarotene cream (0.1%) in combination with betamethasone valerate foam (0.12%) for plaque-type psoriasis. *J Drugs Dermatol* 4: 228–230
21 Bowman PH, Maloney JE, Koo JY (2002) Combination of calcipotriene (Dovonex) ointment and tazarotene (Tazorac) gel *versus* clobetasol ointment in the treatment of plaque psoriasis: a pilot study. *J Am Acad Dermatol* 46: 907–913
22 Koo JY (1998) Tazarotene in combination with phototherapy. *J Am Acad Dermatol* 39: S144–148
23 Hecker D, Worsley J, Yueh G, Kuroda K, Lebwohl M (1999) Interactions between tazarotene and ultraviolet light. *J Am Acad Dermatol* 41: 927–930
24 Koo JY, Lowe NJ, Lew-Kaya DA, Vasilopoulos AI, Lue JC, Sefton J, Gibson JR (2000) Tazarotene plus UVB phototherapy in the treatment of psoriasis. *J Am Acad Dermatol* 43: 821–828
25 Behrens S, Grundmann-Kollmann M, Schiener R, Peter RU, Kerscher M (2000) Combination phototherapy of psoriasis with narrow-band UVB irradiation and topical tazarotene gel. *J Am Acad Dermatol* 42: 493–495
26 Lebwohl M, Ali S (2001) Treatment of psoriasis. Part 1. Topical therapy and phototherapy. *J Am Acad Dermatol* 45: 487–498; quiz 499–502
27 Behrens S, Grundmann-Kollmann M, Peter RU, Kerscher M (1999) Combination treatment of psoriasis with photochemotherapy and tazarotene gel, a receptor-selective topical retinoid. *Br J Dermatol* 141: 177
28 Tzaneva S, Honigsmann H, Tanew A, Seeber A (2002) A comparison of psoralen plus ultraviolet A (PUVA) monotherapy, tacalcitol plus PUVA and tazarotene plus PUVA in patients with chronic plaque-type psoriasis. *Br J Dermatol* 147: 748–753
29 Simpson D, Noble S (2005) Tacrolimus ointment: a review of its use in atopic dermatitis and its clinical potential in other inflammatory skin conditions. *Drugs* 65: 827–858
30 Grassberger M, Baumruker T, Enz A, Hiestand P, Hultsch T, Kalthoff F, Schuler W, Schulz M, Werner FJ, Winiski A et al. (1999) A novel anti-inflammatory drug, SDZ ASM 981, for the treatment of skin diseases: *in vitro* pharmacology. *Br J Dermatol* 141: 264–273
31 de Paulis A, Cirillo R, Ciccarelli A, de Crescenzo G, Oriente A, Marone G (1991) Characterization of the anti-inflammatory effect of FK-506 on human mast cells. *J Immunol* 147: 4278–4285
32 Hultsch T, Muller KD, Meingassner JG, Grassberger M, Schopf RE, Knop J (1998) Ascomycin macrolactam derivative SDZ ASM 981 inhibits the release of granule-associated mediators and of newly synthesized cytokines in RBL 2H3 mast cells in an immunophilin-dependent manner. *Arch Dermatol Res* 290: 501–507
33 Inoue T, Katoh N, Kishimoto S (2006) Prolonged topical application of tacrolimus inhibits immediate hypersensitivity reactions by reducing degranulation of mast cells. *Acta Derm Venereol* 86: 13–16
34 Soter NA, Fleischer AB Jr, Webster GF, Monroe E, Lawrence I (2001) Tacrolimus ointment for the treatment of atopic dermatitis in adult patients: part II, safety. *J Am Acad Dermatol* 44: S39–46
35 Kempers S, Boguniewicz M, Carter E, Jarratt M, Pariser D, Stewart D, Stiller M, Tschen E, Chon K, Wisseh S et al. (2004) A randomized investigator-blinded study comparing pimecrolimus cream 1% with tacrolimus ointment 0.03% in the treatment of pediatric patients with moderate

atopic dermatitis. *J Am Acad Dermatol* 51: 515–525

36 Paller AS, Lebwohl M, Fleischer AB Jr, Antaya R, Langley RG, Kirsner RS, Blum RR, Rico MJ, Jaracz E, Crowe A et al. (2005) Tacrolimus ointment is more effective than pimecrolimus cream with a similar safety profile in the treatment of atopic dermatitis: results from 3 randomized, comparative studies. *J Am Acad Dermatol* 52: 810–822

37 Draelos Z, Nayak A, Pariser D, Shupack JL, Chon K, Abrams B, Paul CF (2005) Pharmacokinetics of topical calcineurin inhibitors in adult atopic dermatitis: a randomized, investigator-blind comparison. *J Am Acad Dermatol* 53: 602–609

38 Reitamo S, Wollenberg A, Schopf E, Perrot JL, Marks R, Ruzicka T, Christophers E, Kapp A, Lahfa M, Rubins A et al. (2000) Safety and efficacy of 1 year of tacrolimus ointment monotherapy in adults with atopic dermatitis. The European Tacrolimus Ointment Study Group. *Arch Dermatol* 136: 999–1006

39 Allen A, Siegfried E, Silverman R, Williams ML, Elias PM, Szabo SK, Korman NJ (2001) Significant absorption of topical tacrolimus in 3 patients with Netherton syndrome. *Arch Dermatol* 137: 747–750

40 Message FDA Available at: www.fda.gov/bbs/topics/news/2006/NEW01299.html. Accessed 20 July 2006

41 Berger TG, Duvic M, Van Voorhees AS, VanBeek MJ, Frieden IJ (2006) The use of topical calcineurin inhibitors in dermatology: safety concerns. Report of the American Academy of Dermatology Association Task Force. *J Am Acad Dermatol* 54: 818–823

42 Yarosh DB, Pena AV, Nay SL, Canning MT, Brown DA (2005) Calcineurin inhibitors decrease DNA repair and apoptosis in human keratinocytes following ultraviolet B irradiation. *J Invest Dermatol* 125: 1020–1025

43 Wijnen RM, Ericzon BG, Tiebosch AT, Buurman WA, Groth CG, Kootstra G (1992) Toxicology of FK506 in the cynomolgus monkey: a clinical, biochemical, and histopathological study. *Transpl Int* 5 Suppl 1: S454–458

44 Novartis F FDA Briefing Statements. Pediatric Advisory Committee Meeting of the US Food and Drug Administration (2005) http://www.fda.gov.ohrms/dockets/ac/05/briefig/2005–4089b2.html

45 Hultsch T, Kapp A, Spergel J (2005) Immunomodulation and safety of topical calcineurin inhibitors for the treatment of atopic dermatitis. *Dermatology* 211: 174–187

46 Lebwohl M, Gower T (2006) A safety assessment of topical calcineurin inhibitors in the treatment of atopic dermatitis. *MedGenMed* 8: 8

47 Bieber T, Cork M, Ellis C, Girolomoni G, Groves R, Langley R, Luger T, Meurer M, Murrell D, Orlow S et al. (2005) Consensus statement on the safety profile of topical calcineurin inhibitors. *Dermatology* 211: 77–78

48 Spergel JM, Leung DY (2006) Safety of topical calcineurin inhibitors in atopic dermatitis: evaluation of the evidence. *Curr Allergy Asthma Rep* 6: 270–274

49 Kainz A, Harabacz I, Cowlrick IS, Gadgil SD, Hagiwara D (2000) Review of the course and outcome of 100 pregnancies in 84 women treated with tacrolimus. *Transplantation* 70: 1718–1721

50 Paul C, Cork M, Rossi AB, Papp KA, Barbier N, de Prost Y (2006) Safety and tolerability of 1% pimecrolimus cream among infants: experience with 1133 patients treated for up to 2 years. *Pediatrics* 117: e118–128

51 Steele JA, Choi C, Kwong PC (2005) Topical tacrolimus in the treatment of inverse psoriasis in children. *J Am Acad Dermatol* 53: 713–716

52 Zonneveld IM, Rubins A, Jablonska S, Dobozy A, Ruzicka T, Kind P, Dubertret L, Bos JD (1998) Topical tacrolimus is not effective in chronic plaque psoriasis. A pilot study. *Arch Dermatol* 134: 1101–1102

53 Remitz A, Reitamo S, Erkko P, Granlund H, Lauerma AI (1999) Tacrolimus ointment improves psoriasis in a microplaque assay. *Br J Dermatol* 141: 103–107

54 Reitamo S, Rissanen J, Remitz A, Granlund H, Erkko P, Elg P, Autio P, Lauerma AI (1998) Tacrolimus ointment does not affect collagen synthesis: results of a single-center randomized trial. *J Invest Dermatol* 111: 396–398

55 Queille-Roussel C, Paul C, Duteil L, Lefebvre MC, Rapatz G, Zagula M, Ortonne JP (2001) The new topical ascomycin derivative SDZ ASM 981 does not induce skin atrophy when applied to normal skin for 4 weeks: a randomized, double-blind controlled study. *Br J Dermatol* 144: 507–513

56 Freeman AK, Linowski GJ, Brady C, Lind L, Vanveldhuisen P, Singer G, Lebwohl M (2003) Tacrolimus ointment for the treatment of psoriasis on the face and intertriginous areas. *J Am Acad*

Dermatol 48: 564–568
57 Yamamoto T, Nishioka K (2000) Topical tacrolimus is effective for facial lesions of psoriasis. *Acta Derm Venereol* 80: 451
58 Yamamoto T, Nishioka K (2003) Topical tacrolimus: an effective therapy for facial psoriasis. *Eur J Dermatol* 13: 471–473
59 Lebwohl M, Freeman AK, Chapman MS, Feldman SR, Hartle JE, Henning A (2004) Tacrolimus ointment is effective for facial and intertriginous psoriasis. *J Am Acad Dermatol* 51: 723–730
60 Nagao K, Ishiko A, Yokoyama T, Tanikawa A, Amagai M (2003) A case of generalized pustular psoriasis treated with topical tacrolimus. *Arch Dermatol* 139: 1219
61 Ortonne JP, van de Kerkhof PC, Prinz JC, Bieber T, Lahfa M, Rubins A, Wozel G, Lorette G (2006) 0.3% Tacrolimus gel and 0.5% Tacrolimus cream show efficacy in mild to moderate plaque psoriasis: Results of a randomized, open-label, observer-blinded study. *Acta Derm Venereol* 86: 29–33
62 Mrowietz U, Graeber M, Brautigam M, Thurston M, Wagenaar A, Weidinger G, Christophers E (1998) The novel ascomycin derivative SDZ ASM 981 is effective for psoriasis when used topically under occlusion. *Br J Dermatol* 139: 992–996
63 Gribetz C, Ling M, Lebwohl M, Pariser D, Draelos Z, Gottlieb AB, Zaias N, Chen DM, Parneix-Spake A, Hultsch T et al. (2004) Pimecrolimus cream 1% in the treatment of intertriginous psoriasis: a double-blind, randomized study. *J Am Acad Dermatol* 51: 731–738
64 Mrowietz U, Wustlich S, Hoexter G, Graeber M, Brautigam M, Luger T (2003) An experimental ointment formulation of pimecrolimus is effective in psoriasis without occlusion. *Acta Derm Venereol* 83: 351–353
65 Ormerod AD, Shah SA, Copeland P, Omar G, Winfield A (2005) Treatment of psoriasis with topical sirolimus: preclinical development and a randomized, double-blind trial. *Br J Dermatol* 152: 758–764
66 Carroll CL, Clarke J, Camacho F, Balkrishnan R, Feldman SR (2005) Topical tacrolimus ointment combined with 6% salicylic acid gel for plaque psoriasis treatment. *Arch Dermatol* 141: 43–46
67 Everett MA, Daffer E, Coffey CM (1961) Coal tar and ultraviolet light. *Arch Dermatol* 84: 473–476
68 Goeckerman W (1925) Treatment of psoriasis. *Northwest Med* 24: 229–231
69 Stoughton RB, DeQuoy P, Walter JF (1978) Crude coal tar plus near ultraviolet light suppresses DNA synthesis in epidermis. *Arch Dermatol* 114: 43–45
70 Goeckerman W (1931) Treatment of psoriasis. Continued observations on the use of crude coal tar and ultraviolet light. *Arch Dermatol Syphilol* 30: 446–450
71 Lee E, Koo J (2005) Modern modified 'ultra' Goeckerman therapy: a PASI assessment of a very effective therapy for psoriasis resistant to both prebiologic and biologic therapies. *J Dermatolog Treat* 16: 102–107
72 Koo J, Lebwohl M (1999) Duration of remission of psoriasis therapies. *J Am Acad Dermatol* 41: 51–59
73 Goodfield M, Kownacki S, Berth-Jones J (2004) Double-blind, randomised, multicentre, parallel group study comparing a 1% coal tar preparation (Exorex) with a 5% coal tar preparation (Alphosyl) in chronic plaque psoriasis. *J Dermatolog Treat* 15: 14–22
74 Lin AN, Moses K (1985) Tar revisited. *Int J Dermatol* 24: 216–218
75 Sharma V, Kaur I, Kumar B (2003) Calcipotriol *versus* coal tar: a prospective randomized study in stable plaque psoriasis. *Int J Dermatol* 42: 834–838
76 Thami GP, Sarkar R (2002) Coal tar: past, present and future. *Clin Exp Dermatol* 27: 99–103
77 Silverman A, Menter A, Hairston JL (1995) Tars and anthralins. *Dermatol Clin* 13: 817–833
78 McGill A, Frank A, Emmett N, Turnbull DM, Birch-Machin MA, Reynolds NJ (2005) The anti-psoriatic drug anthralin accumulates in keratinocyte mitochondria, dissipates mitochondrial membrane potential, and induces apoptosis through a pathway dependent on respiratory competent mitochondria. *Faseb J* 19: 1012–1014
79 Mahrle G (1997) Dithranol. *Clin Dermatol* 15: 723–737
80 Ashton RE, Andre P, Lowe NJ, Whitefield M (1983) Anthralin: historical and current perspectives. *J Am Acad Dermatol* 9: 173–192
81 Lebwohl M, Abel E, Zanolli M, Koo J, Drake L (1995) Topical therapy for psoriasis. *Int J Dermatol* 34: 673–684
82 Harris DR (1998) Old wine in new bottles: the revival of anthralin. *Cutis* 62: 201–203
83 Schaefer H, Farber EM, Goldberg L, Schalla W (1980) Limited application period for dithranol in

psoriasis. Preliminary report on penetration and clinical efficacy. *Br J Dermatol* 102: 571–573
84 Marsden JR, Coburn PR, Marks J, Shuster S (1983) Measurement of the response of psoriasis to short-term application of anthralin. *Br J Dermatol* 109: 209–218
85 Volden G, Bjornberg A, Tegner E, Pedersen NB, Arles UB, Agren S, Brolund L (1992) Short-contact treatment at home with Micanol. *Acta Derm Venereol Suppl (Stockh)* 172: 20–22
86 Ramsay B, Lawrence CM, Bruce JM, Shuster S (1990) The effect of triethanolamine application on anthralin-induced inflammation and therapeutic effect in psoriasis. *J Am Acad Dermatol* 23: 73–76
87 Endzweig-Gribetz CH, Brady C, Lynde C, Sibbald D, Lebwohl M (2002) Drug interactions in psoriasis: the pros and cons of combining topical psoriasis therapies. *J Cutan Med Surg* 6: 12–16
88 Muller R, Naumann E, Detmar M, Orfanos CE (1987) Stability of cignolin (dithranol) in ointments containing tar with and without the addition of salicylic acid. Oxidation to danthron and dithranol dimer. *Hautarzt* 38: 107–111
89 Lebwohl M (1999) The role of salicylic acid in the treatment of psoriasis. *Int J Dermatol* 38: 16–24
90 Huber C, Christophers E (1977) "Keratolytic" effect of salicylic acid. *Arch Dermatol Res* 257: 293–297
91 Davies M, Marks R (1976) Studies on the effect of salicylic acid on normal skin. *Br J Dermatol* 95: 187–192
92 Krochmal L, Wang JC, Patel B, Rodgers J (1989) Topical corticosteroid compounding: effects on physicochemical stability and skin penetration rate. *J Am Acad Dermatol* 21: 979–984
93 Hovding G (1981) Treatment of psoriasis of the scalp with betamethasone 17, 21-dipropionate plus salicylic acid lotion ('Diprosalic'). *Pharmatherapeutica* 3: 61–66
94 Koo J, Cuffie CA, Tanner DJ, Bressinck R, Cornell RC, DeVillez RL, Edwards L, Breneman DL, Piacquadio DJ, Guzzo CA et al. (1998) Mometasone furoate 0.1%-salicylic acid 5% ointment *versus* mometasone furoate 0.1% ointment in the treatment of moderate-to-severe psoriasis: a multicenter study. *Clin Ther* 20: 283–291
95 Lebwohl M, Menter A, Koo J, Feldman SR (2004) Combination therapy to treat moderate to severe psoriasis. *J Am Acad Dermatol* 50: 416–430
96 Proudfoot AT (1983) Toxicity of salicylates. *Am J Med* 75: 99–103

Treatment of Psoriasis
Edited by J.M. Weinberg

Ultraviolet and laser therapy

Rahat S. Azfar and Abby S. Van Voorhees

Department of Dermatology, University of Pennsylvania, 3600 Spruce St, 2 Maloney, Philadelphia, PA 19104, USA

Introduction

Natural sunlight's beneficial effect on psoriasis has been long known. This observation led over the past century to the utilization of artificial light sources for the treatment of psoriasis. For over seven decades, phototherapy using artificial ultraviolet light has been an established standard in the treatment of psoriasis. Advancements in our understanding of ultraviolet energy and photobiology have led to a number of available modalities in this field. After a brief historical introduction, we will discuss these techniques in detail, with emphasis on indications, efficacy, advantages and disadvantages and administration of each modality.

Broadband UVB phototherapy first began in the 1920s in combination with topical medication [1]. Chemotherapeutic adjuncts were first described by Goeckerman in 1925 when he introduced rough coal tar as a photosensitizer for sunlight. Prior to this however, a progenitor of anthralin, a natural product called chrysarobin found in Goa powder and derived from the South American araroba tree was used in the treatment of psoriasis beginning in the mid 19th century. While the synthesis of anthralin occurred in 1916, in 1953 it was substituted by Ingram into the Goeckerman protocol [2, 3].

Balneophototherapy, the combined treatment of ultraviolet therapy and salt water baths, was formally introduced as a therapeutic modality in Israel in the 1950s after patients reported an improvement of their psoriasis at the Dead Sea. The ambient light at this low altitude is considered less erythemogenic and offers greater efficacy than ambient sunlight elsewhere. This phenomenon then led to the development of balneophototherapy centers in Germany in the 1970s [4].

Photochemotherapy using psoralens to enhance the efficacy of ultraviolet A light (320–400 nm) as pUVA therapy was also introduced in the 1970s. Oral pUVA therapy was developed in 1972 by Mortazawi for the treatment of psoriasis and popularized in 1974 by Parrish and Fitzpatrick et al. [5]. This was followed in 1975 by Mortazawi and Obertse-Lehn's introduction of topical pUVA and by the development of bath pUVA in 1977 by Born [3].

While broadband ultraviolet light (bbUVB) (290–320 nm) phototherapy has been used since the early part of the 20th Century, targeted emission spectra were pioneered in Europe by Fischer in 1976, which resulted in the development of narrowband UVB. But it was not until 1998 that narrowband therapy was introduced to North America [6]. Over time, there has been a shift from hot quartz lamps to fluorescent tubes such as the Philips TL-01 for delivery of this modality, allowing for a more precise emission [4].

The excited dimer, or excimer laser has been used in multiple areas of medicine. Application of the xenon-chloride excimer laser, with a wavelength of 308 nm, was first described as an effective antipsoriatic therapy in 1997 by Bonis [7]. Other laser systems such as the flashlamp pulse dye laser (PDL, 585 nm) were described in the 1990s by Hacker and Rasmussen [8].

The combination of lights with systemic medications has been studied since the 1980s. In particular, the combination of systemic retinoids and UVB or pUVA has demonstrated efficacy and offers significant advantages in the management of psoriasis. Finally, data describing the combination of light therapy with the latest weapons in the psoriasis arsenal, the 'biologics', have started to emerge in the early years of this new Century.

Ultraviolet B

The mechanism of action of UVB light is not yet fully elucidated. UVB is absorbed mainly in the epidermis. It inhibits DNA synthesis and epidermal keratinocyte hyperproliferation, and induces T cell apoptosis and immunosuppressive and anti-inflammatory cytokines [6]. High dose UVB induces intermediate apoptosis through activation of cell death receptors, whereas lower doses of UVB can produce programmed cell death via DNA damage.

Ultraviolet B light treatment is indicated for patients with moderate or severe disease. Contraindications include known photosensitivity, either secondary to a photosensitive disease such as xeroderma pigmentosum, lupus or polymorphous light eruption, or secondary to photosensitizing medications.

Side effects of UVB include erythema, burns, and photodamage. Erythema from UVB exposure is produced within 12–15 h for narrowband UVB (nbUVB) and 8–12 h for broadband UVB. The risk of burning with either modality is less than with pUVA, however.

Broadband UVB versus *narrowband UVB*

Although embraced more quickly in Europe, targeted ultraviolet B treatment around the 311 nm spectrum using fluorescent Philips TL-01 lamps has been more slowly accepted in North America. Narrowband therapy is more expensive than broadband secondary to the cost of the machines. Narrowband bulbs need more frequent replacement, with fluences decreasing more quickly than with traditional broadband ultraviolet bulbs. It also requires longer treatment time, i.e., longer standing in the booth, and higher energies to achieve the same level of erythema than bbUVB [4, 9, 10].

On the other hand, advantages of nbUVB therapy include fewer phototoxic and photoallergic drug reactions, faster response and greater efficacy in patients with severe disease and varying skin types [4, 11, 12]. Finally, nbUVB may have a greater immunomodulatory effect than bbUVB and act more through local rather than systemic effects [13].

Another theoretical advantage may be that perhaps the smaller spectrum of UVB is less carcinogenic than bbUVB. However, there is a paucity of data comparing the two modalities in humans. Murine models have thus far shown conflicting results [14]. Furthermore, a recent retrospective study of psoriatic patients who were followed for 533- and 726- person years after receiving broadband and narrowband therapy, respectively, did not find any cases of skin cancer attributable to either therapy [15]. In a subsequent group of 1'908 patients followed for a median of 4 years after treatment with narrowband for psoriasis and other conditions, a small and statistically insignificant adjusted risk of increased basal cell cancer was reported [16]. Neither study has sufficient data on the skin types of their subjects. Furthermore, a systematic review on UVB (not specific for narrow- or broadband) phototherapy and the risk of skin cancer from 1966 to 2002 reported an overwhelmingly negative risk for skin cancer [17]. Nonetheless, current guidelines suggest regular monitoring of patients considered at risk for skin cancer, particularly those with skin types I or II and blonde or red hair [18].

Another area lacking in comparative data between narrowband and broadband UVB is duration of remission. In two separate studies performed by the same investigators, relapse free rates in patients who received narrowband UVB were 38% [19] *versus* 5% in patients who received bbUVB after one year [20].

Data on relative frequency and severity of burning with narrowband and broadband phototherapy are mixed, with studies reporting fewer, equal and greater numbers of burning episodes [14]. Coven et al., however, have noted a correlation between a greater and longer erythema response and higher frequency of sunburn cells in patients receiving 2.0 MED in patients receiving nbUVB *versus* bbUVB in their head to head analysis [11].

Administration of broadband ultraviolet therapy

Protocols for administration of broadband phototherapy vary by center. In general, dosing may be determined by minimal erythema dose (MED) or skin type. If an MED is determined, then the patient's treatment is begun with exposures at 50–100% of the MED.

Subsequent dosing regimens can be based on erythemogenic or nonerythemogenic schedules, with maximal results produced from light near the patient's MED. Thus, the major advantage to using an erythemogenic schedule is better efficacy, whereas a nonerythemogenic schedule will reduce the risks of burn and patient discomfort and ought to theoretically minimize the cumulative dose. Generally doses are increased by 10–25% of the prior treatment dose.

An alternative initial dosing strategy utilizing skin type is also frequently followed. Once the initial dose is determined, the amount of UVB is increased incrementally until the MED is reached. The patient is subsequently maintained at just below MED.

Treatment with both approaches is given 3–5 times weekly. 15–25 treatments are usually needed to achieve skin clearance.

Administration of narrowband ultraviolet therapy

Here again protocols vary by center. Similar to broadband therapy, initial dosing can be based on MED or on skin type as described above.

If using the MED approach, treatments are generally begun at 50–70% of the MED and subsequently increased by 10–20% of the MED. Suberythemogenic doses are preferred, as with just slightly more treatments, equivalent efficacy is achieved as with near-erythemogenic dosing [14, 21].

Treatments are usually given three times weekly with narrowband UVB as well [22, 23]. However, in some cases, even twice weekly treatments may be adequate as noted in a study of Asian skin types III–V using varied exposure increments [24].

Clearance is achieved in approximately 63–80% of patients [6]. Although responses are generally more rapid with nbUVB than with broadband, 15–20 treatments are required to achieve greater than 50% disease improvement. Once clearance is achieved, maintenance therapy once weekly is an option.

UVB and topicals

Bland emollients

Emollients are commonly used in conjunction with phototherapy to moisturize the skin and to reduce the itching and dryness often associated with phototherapy. Emollients can also alter the ultraviolet transmission of skin. While some emollients have photoprotective properties which can reduce the efficacy of phototherapy, others can also reduce back scatter of radiation from plaques, thus enhancing light absorption [25]. The optimal emollient is one that is non-photosensitizing and non-UV absorbing. An oil-in-water type emollient used in conjunction with broadband ultraviolet B phototherapy produced a greater therapeutic effect on psoriatic plaques than broadband UVB alone [26]. Similarly, mineral oil applied to lesions 5 mins before entering a narrowband UVB booth helps improve skin's refractive index, allowing enhanced UVB penetration, and thus increasing the efficacy of treatment over narrowband therapy alone [27]. There are no known side effects from mineral oil pretreatment.

Keratolytics and ultraviolet B therapy

Keratolytics such as salicylic acid are useful in diminishing thick scale from psoriatic plaques, which would otherwise scatter light. Concentrations of up to 10% are commonly used. However, improvement in efficacy needs to be balanced with the inherent light absorptive capabilities of salicylic acid. If used immediately before ultraviolet B light therapy, salicylic acid may increase the minimal erythema dose of UVB light [28–30]. It is therefore recommended that keratolytics be applied after light treatment, or if used prior to treatment, be washed off completely. For patients who cannot tolerate the irritation from salicylic acid, lactic acid may also be utilized to diminish scaling.

Goeckerman therapy

Much of our knowledge of ultraviolet B phototherapy stems from greater than 60 years of experience with Goeckerman treatments. Since its introduction, many variations of the Goeckerman regimen and its components have been studied. Today, the traditional inpatient Goeckerman regimen has been successfully modified to be delivered as an outpatient daycare treatment [31, 32]. Moreover, therapy has evolved to include other agents such as salicylic acid, anthralin, acitretin, tazarotene, and calcipotriene [33].

Both the crude coal tar and ultraviolet B radiation used in this regimen are thought to have independent and additive beneficial effects [34, 35]. Tar appears to suppress DNA synthesis when used in conjunction with suberythemogenic doses of UVB to the same levels as erythemogenic UVB alone. This results in less potential for burning and irritation than with erythemogenic UVB doses [36, 37].

Menter and Cram showed that the average duration of treatment to achieve >90% skin clearance was 18 days, with 90% clearance rates at 8 months and 73% clearance rates at 1 year [38]. In a recent report, 25 out of 25 patients admitted for Goeckerman therapy achieved PASI 75 at 3 months, with 96% reaching PASI 75 after 2 months, and with most patients discharged after 1–2 months [33]. Treatment with home Goeckerman therapy however yields 5 months of remission [39]. Although practiced, no controlled studies have specifically reported on the efficacy of tar and narrowband light. Currently, tar is applied for at least 4 h daily at least five times a week, after exposure to ultraviolet B light.

Debates on the long-term safety of Goeckerman treatment have been ongoing. Chromosomal aberrations in peripheral lymphocytes were recently reported in patients undergoing inpatient Goeckerman treatment with ultraviolet B therapy [40]. Furthermore, the carcinogenic potentiation of light and tar has been demonstrated *in vitro* and in animal models [41]. However tar as used in the Goeckerman technique was not found to be carcinogenic in psoriatic patients in a 25 year follow-up study done at Mayo clinic [42]. Finally, although highly efficacious, limitations to Goeckerman treatment include the excessive daily time commitment required by this modality. Furthermore, few day treatment centers remain in the US.

Ingram method

Although the exact mechanism of action is unclear, the Ingram method entailed a daily tar bath, broadband ultraviolet radiation, followed by application of a stiff paste of dithranol or anthralin in a daycare or hospital setting. In the recent past, short contact therapy with an up to 2 h application of dithranol was shown to be just as effective [43]. Minimizing treatment time with dithranol reduces both the irritancy and staining associated with dithranol [44]. Moreover, reducing short contact treatment with dithranol to three times weekly in conjunction with five times weekly broadband light is as effective as five times a week treatment with dithranol and broadband UVB light. Furthermore, Ingram therapy with narrowband light has been demonstrated to be at least as effective as that with broadband UVB [45]. Other modifications include the use of dithranol in a cream base with salicylic acid to increase the keratolytic effect of the treatment.

Conflicting information exists on whether the combination of ultraviolet B, tar and anthralin *versus* anthralin alone produces prolonged remission or improves treatment efficacy [46–48]. Ultimately however, the relatively modest advantages of Ingram therapy in combination with the limited availability of anthralin, the inconvenience of application, and the associated erythema and swelling lessen the utility of this approach.

Tazarotene and UVB

Tazarotene has antiproliferative effects, normalizes altered keratinocyte differentiation, and decreases dermal and epidermal inflammation [49]. In a recent review of retinoid therapy in psoriasis, a non-statistically significant reduction in cumulative dose and time to achieve 50% efficacy in patients treated with combination therapy with tazarotene gel *versus* broadband ultraviolet monotherapy was noted [50]. In addition, in an intrapatient controlled study of tazarotene and narrowband ultraviolet light *versus* nbUVB alone, 64% PASI reduction was achieved with the intervention and 48% in the control group respectively at 4 weeks. Neither significant irritation from tazarotene or phototoxicity from the light therapy were seen [49]. Tazarotene can cause photosensitivity, and as it is a teratogen, it is contraindicated in pregnancy and in women not using adequate contraception. Its additive value therefore in combination with UVB phototherapy remains uncertain. When utilized it is generally applied after light treatments.

Vitamin D derivatives and UVB

Vitamin D derivatives including calcipotriene (known as calcipotriol outside the US), calcitriol, maxacalcitol and tacalcitol have been used in numerous studies with ultraviolet B phototherapy. These analogs downregulate cell proliferation, induce keratinocyte differentiation, and have immunomodulatory effects [51, 52]. Whereas improved efficacy using combination therapy with topical vitamin D derivatives and either narrowband or broadband UVB *versus* calcipotriene alone or UVB alone has been reported in a number of studies [53–58], a systematic review of randomized controlled trials evaluating such regimens showed only a small and clinically insignificant enhancement in efficacy [59]. Instead, the benefit of combining the two modalities may lie in reducing the overall exposure to ultraviolet light, hence reducing the risks associated with narrow- or broadband UVB phototherapy and providing greater patient convenience with fewer phototherapy sessions [60–62].

Calcipotriene and the other vitamin D derivatives are usually applied once to twice daily and accompanied by three times weekly UVB phototherapy. Because of reports of an immediate burning sensation with UVB phototherapy when followed by immediate application of calcipotriol [63], application is recommended 2–3 h before or after UVB exposure. Topical calcitriol is degraded by ultraviolet light [64]. A thin layer of calcipotriene on the other hand, is not significantly degraded by UVB [65]. Other adverse effects include skin irritation, which usually improves with time, hyperpigmentation, and a risk of hypercalcemia if the topical vitamin D analog is applied to large surface areas over a long period of time, particularly in patients with preexisting renal insufficiency. Additionally, caution is advised when initiating the topical adjunct in patients already receiving phototherapy as cases of increased photosensitivity have been described [66].

Corticosteroids and UVB

Although these two modalities exert beneficial effects on psoriasis, six out of seven studies using the combination of ultraviolet B phototherapy and topical steroids showed lack of an additive benefit [67]. To the contrary, this combination may reduce the duration of remission although it is commonly used [68].

Balneophototherapy

Although the mechanism of action of balneophototherapy is not fully elucidated, it is hypothesized to exert its effects through chemical, thermal, and immunologic modulation of the skin. There is no standard protocol. A number of specialized areas in the world exist, where natural mineral waters are utilized with natural light exposure to treat psoriasis, such as the Dead Sea in Israel, the Kangal hot spring in Turkey, and the Blue Lagoon in Iceland [69]. Furthermore, balneophototherapy centers utilizing artificial ultraviolet light in combination with mineralized water exist in many European countries.

Balneophototherapy has been shown to produce histologic normalization of the epidermis, reduction in epidermal hyperproliferative markers and reduction of epidermal and dermal T cell populations [70, 71]. It has demonstrated efficacy in guttate and plaque type psoriasis [72]. 48–70% of patients are reported to achieve complete remission, with the average duration of remission being 3–6 months [73, 74]. Recurrences are experienced in 41–45% of patients at 1 month [39]. Like with other forms of UVB therapy risks of chronic balneophototherapy include photodamage and skin cancer [75]. More acutely, transient pruritis and stinging can occur. Efficacy of balneophototherapy relative to narrowband phototherapy has been demonstrated to be nearly equivalent. Dawe et al. showed only a marginal benefit in clearance of lesions with Dead Sea Salt soaks with nbUVB than with nbUVB alone [76]. Similarly, phototherapy with French saline spa water showed comparable efficacy to narrowband ultraviolet alone for localized lesions [74].

Home UVB

Although home ultraviolet B phototherapy was introduced in the late 1970s [77], no randomized trials have been done evaluating its efficacy. Most studies have utilized broadband ultraviolet B light. Protocols for home treatment with narrowband bulbs have been developed however [78]. Candidates for home phototherapy are those who are intelligent, compliant, motivated and have prior experience with ultraviolet light for whom a regular schedule of office-based treatment is not feasible for logistic reasons. Benefits of home ultraviolet B phototherapy include decreased time, travel and cost to the patient [79]. Concerns among practitioners regarding medicolegal liability, lack of medical supervision and poor service and equipment are common [80, 81].

UVB and systemics

Oral retinoids and ultraviolet B

The combination of acitretin with ultraviolet B phototherapy produces synergistic results, allowing for lower cumulative doses of UVB. Retinoids cause thinning of the stratum corneum and epidermis, which leads to increased sensitivity to ultraviolet light.

In a double-blind placebo-controlled randomized multicenter trial of patients with severe psoriasis comparing low dose acitretin (25–35 mg) combined with broadband UV-B irradiation *versus* placebo and broadband UVB, 60% of patients achieved 75% or greater improvement in the psoriasis severity index with the combination treatment whereas only 24% of the controls did. The median cumulative UV-B dose required to achieve this level of response was significantly lower, 6.9 J/cm^2 in the combination group *versus* 11.8 J/cm^2 in the control. No difference was seen in side effects [82]. Similarly, Iest and Boer reported 89% of their patients treated with acitretin and broadband UVB achieved 80–100% clearance while 62.5% of those receiving bbUVB only cleared by the same criteria. Furthermore those treated with acitretin and UVB required significantly fewer phototherapy sessions than those receiving phototherapy alone [83]. Lowe et al. also found that patients treated with a combination of broadband UVB and 50 mg daily of acitretin for 3 months showed 74% improvement *versus* 35% improvement in those receiving UVB with placebo *versus* 42% in those receiving acitretin alone, with the intervention group requiring significantly lower total UVB treatment time and cumulative UVB dose to achieve the superior results [84].

No prospective trial data has yet to be published on acitretin combined with narrowband UVB phototherapy. Nevertheless, existing reports suggest that this combination is as synergistically useful as acitretin and broadband UVB. A retrospective study of 40 severe psoriasis patients demonstrated a PASI 75 response in 72.5% receiving treatment with acitretin and NB-UVB [85]. Furthermore a multi-tier trial comparing narrowband UVB alone *versus* etretinate (the parent compound of acitretin) with NB-UVB, and etretinate with pUVA demonstrated that the retinoid NB-UVB combination was effective at achieving clearance in 93% of patients. The total number of joules was also greatly diminished compared with patients receiving NB-UVB treatments alone (8 J/cm^2 *versus* 12.7 J/cm^2) [86]. The combination of narrowband ultraviolet phototherapy with acitretin has been reported to be efficacious in the treatment of severe pustular psoriasis of von Zumbusch within 10 sessions of phototherapy [87].

Oral retinoid therapy can be begun either before or during the course of UVB therapy as long as the UVB dose is appropriately modified. If the retinoid is added after UVB therapy is in progress, then care should be taken to avoid burning by reducing the dose of light therapy by 30–50% [10]. Alternatively the retinoid can be started about 2 weeks prior to commencing phototherapy, with MED testing performed while the patient is on a stable dose of the oral retinoid.

Side effects of retinoid therapy are minimized when it is used in conjunction with ultraviolet light as lower doses of retinoids are used. Furthermore, since concomitant retinoid therapy allows a significant reduction in the cumulative UVB dose, the risk of long-term adverse effects associated with UVB is theoretically diminished. The true rate of nonmelanoma skin cancer seen with ReUVB is not known. Care in using systemic retinoids in women of childbearing potential is necessary and their use may be contraindicated as these drugs are potent teratogens.

Methotrexate and ultraviolet B

The combination of methotrexate and narrowband light therapy enhances the efficacy of and produces longer remission than narrowband UVB alone. Cumulative doses of both treatments modalities required to achieve remission are lower than when either modality is used alone [88]. In addition to the risks inherent in the individual methods, the erythema recall phenomenon is a possible concern. This however has not been reported in trials evaluating this combination approach [88, 89]. Nonetheless, it is prudent to avoid exposing patients to light for 48–72 h following methotrexate dosing. Furthermore, the risk of skin cancer when using both of these modalities in combination is not known. A 3 week lead-in with methotrexate alone is followed by MED testing and then the addition of narrowband ultraviolet B. As more options for treatment become available, this combination is used less frequently. However where treatment with the other systemic agents presents prohibitive economic obstacles, this combination regimen may prove to be useful.

Psoralen and UVB

Although traditionally used with ultraviolet A light, psoralen has been described as an adjunct to narrowband phototherapy in a limited number of studies. In a randomized trial comparing twice weekly psoralen-narrowband UVB (pUVB) to pUVA therapy, psoralen nUVB was just as effective in clearing patients as pUVA with no significant difference seen in relapse rates at 3 months. Major side effects included erythema, which was noted in equal proportions of patients and one case of blistering within a psoriatic plaque in a pUVB patient [90]. Other groups have also reported similarly successful results with pUVB [91, 92], with a recent small study showing increased benefit when using topical psoralen with narrowband UVB than with nbUVB alone [93]. No long-term safety data exists and the mechanism of action has not been studied.

Cyclosporine and UVB

The use of cyclosporine with ultraviolet light has not been well studied and is contraindicated because of the risk of nonmelanoma skin caner. While there is no data on efficacy or safety of this combination regimen, this combination has been used by some experts for short courses [68]. Monitoring for hypertension as well as for lab abnormalities with use of cyclosporine is indicated. Patients with renal impairment are not candidates for treatment with cyclosporine.

Lasers

Excimer

Excimer lasers produce a coherent wavelength of light at 308 nm that induces T cell depletion, alteration of apoptosis-related molecules, and a decreased proliferation index in psoriatic plaques [94, 95]. Multiple treatment regimens are used including fixed dosing, induration or response-based dosing, and multiple high doses or single high doses. Treatments are generally given two to three times weekly. 69–85% of patients have been reported to achieve a satisfactory response after a mean number of 6–13 treatments, with clearance being achieved faster with higher and more frequent dosing [96]. Advantages of excimer therapy include long remissions of up to 2 years, faster clearance rates in comparison to traditional UVB phototherapy and decreased cumulative doses [96–98]. The excimer laser is effective for localized psoriasis, and can be used for palmoplantar, scalp and inverse disease [99–101]. The use of the excimer system for more diffuse disease is unrealistic. Other issues of concern include pain, focal blistering, and hyperpigmentation, and the potential risk of long-term side effects such as skin cancer.

Pulsed dye

Pulsed dye lasers are capable of penetrating the dermis to a depth of 1.2 mm to photocoagulate vessels up to 100 micrometers in diameter [102]. They can be used to target the increased angiogenesis and vascularity of psoriatic lesions, and also reduce T-lymphocyte proliferation in the papillary dermis [103, 104]. Benefits of this modality include selective tissue targeting, treatment of plaques resistant to topical therapy, and induction of long-term remissions [96, 105, 106]. Response rates have ranged from 57–82% with a proportion of patients completely clearing [96]. Treatments are generally given once every 2–6 weeks. Both long and short pulsewidth treatments have been used, with longer pulsewidths being associated with less pain and purpura and faster healing [103]. Side effects are mostly transient and can include purpura, crusting, hyper and hypopigmentation, and moderate discomfort during treatments.

Ultraviolet A

UVA alone

Very little data exists on the use of UVA alone. Some data in a small number of tanning bed studies show a small beneficial effect in psoriasis [107]. A randomized placebo controlled trial of UVA sunbed therapy for example showed a very small but statistically significant improvement in modified PASI scores of the body halves receiving 99.3% UVA *versus* receiving visible light. No clearing was noted after 12 treatment sessions [108].

pUVA

Ultraviolet A therapy (320–400 nm) is most commonly used in conjunction with psoralen, a naturally occurring plant compound that causes a phototoxic phytophotodermatitis reaction. With an action spectrum of 320–340 nm, psoralen is a lipophilic compound that is poorly absorbed by the gut. The mechanism of action of psoralen photochemotherapy is not fully known. It is known however that psoralen intercalates between DNA base pairs. Upon exposure to ultraviolet A light, it crosslinks with pyrimidine bases, forming cyclobutane rings. Additionally, pUVA therapy induces reactive oxygen formation which cause cell and membrane damage to T-lymphocytes and antigen presenting cells [4, 109]. pUVA also induces delayed apoptosis through DNA damage via a programmed cell death mechanism.

Two types of oral psoralen are available – 8 methoxypsoralen (8-MOP) is used more commonly in the US, whereas Europeans use 5 methoxypsoralen (5-MOP). The newest formulation of 8-MOP, methoxsalen, has greater bioavailability and earlier photosensitization onset time than other psoralens. pUVA is indicated for patients with moderate to severe psoriasis. Photochemotherapy is contraindicated in those patients with a history of xeroderma pigmentosum, lupus erythematosus or other light sensitive diseases, hepatic insufficiency, invasive squamous cell cancer, aphakia, or those who are lactating, pregnant or on warfarin or phenytoin.

Erythema, which varies by individual susceptibility, body site and dose, typically appears 24–48 h after treatment, but may occur up to 96 h post exposure. The dose response curve for erythema is steeper with photochemotherapy than with sunlight or UVB, thus making it relatively easier to produce a painful burn with pUVA. When compared to equally erythemogenic doses of UVB, for example, pUVA induces more dermal vessel damage and greater duration of dermal and epidermal abnormalities. Furthermore, Tanew et al. found that suberythemogenic pUVA doses of 1/2 to 2/3 of the minimal phototoxic dose (MPD) were as efficacious as erythemogenic doses in achieving clearance, while reducing the cumulative UVA dose received [110]. Thus, every effort should be made to use the lowest dose feasible. In addition, pretreatment and yearly ophthalmologic examinations and protective eyewear are necessary preventative measures against the risk of cataract development with systemic therapy. Other side effects include CNS effects such as nervousness, vertigo, fatigue, depression, dizziness, headache, and malaise as well as pruritis, photoaging, nausea and an increased risk of nonmelanoma skin cancer after 200 treatments [111]. Relative to 8-MOP, 5-methoxysoralen is less likely to produce gastrointestinal side effects. Other disadvantages of oral pUVA include the inconvenience of wearing protective eyewear.

A meta-analysis of eight large studies with at least 5 year follow up of patients receiving pUVA showed that the overall incidence of squamous cell carcinoma was 14 times higher in those patients receiving 200 or more treatments in comparison to those patients receiving less than 100 pUVA treatments. The same analysis showed that patients in the high treatment number group had a 3:1 ratio of SCC to basal cell carcinomas whereas patients receiving less than 100 treatments were more apt to have BCCs than SCCs [112]. Additionally, there is a dose dependent increased risk of genital squamous cell cancers in men, whose genitalia was initially not shielded during photochemotherapy, which is persistent even after shielding has occurred with later sessions [113, 114].

Stern et al. reported a nearly six-fold increased adjusted risk of melanoma 15 years after first pUVA treatment in their cohort of patients. The risk appears to increase with time and may be greater in patients receiving greater than 200 pUVA treatment [115]. This data on melanoma risk must be interpreted with caution however, as other groups have failed to find a significant increase of melanoma incidence in their pUVA treated patients [116]. No increased risk of melanoma or nonmelanoma skin cancer has been reported for topical photochemotherapies [117, 118]. Finally, a large cohort of Swedish patients who received photochemotherapy, including both systemic and topical formulations, for psoriasis as well as other indications did not show an increased risk of melanoma after an average of 16 years of follow-up [119].

Photochemotherapy is highly effective in clearing most types of psoriasis, with 70–90% of patients achieving partial or complete remission [6]. 42% of patients are clear for over 1 year, with the average duration of remission being 64 weeks. With the addition of once weekly to once every 2 or 3 week maintenance therapy, even longer remissions can be produced [39].

Topical variations of pUVA therapy include baths, soaks, creams, and lotions. Unlike the pills, these lack systemic effects such as nausea or CNS disturbance and cataract risk, and can be used for localized therapy. Like its oral equivalent, bath photochemotherapy inhibits epidermal cell proliferation and decreases T lymphocyte activity [120]. Response rates between topical and oral pUVA are similar, with clearance achieved with the same number of treatments yet requiring three to six times lower doses with bath treatment compared to oral. Of note, photosensitivity with bath pUVA dissipates faster than oral pUVA [121, 122]. Yet there is a greater tendency to burn with bath pUVA in comparison to oral therapy.

Administration of pUVA

An individual's minimal phototoxic dose, or MPD, is defined as the lowest dose of UVA that causes erythema after exposure to psoralen. While the MPD can be determined and used as a basis for pUVA treatments, in general pUVA is based on skin type. If used, the MPD is determined prior to the commencement of photochemotherapy. For oral photochemotherapy, treatment is begun at UVA doses at 70% of this dose. Oral 8-methoxypsoralen is given 1.5 h before exposure of ultraviolet light. The medication is available in 10 mg capsules and dose is determined according to a patient's weight [123]. 5-methoxypsoralen is given at 1.2 mg/kg 2 h before light exposure. Therapy is generally given two to three times weekly on nonconsecutive days [123].

Optimal treatment protocols based on controlled trials for bath and other types of topical pUVA therapy have not yet been established. Generally, bath photochemotherapy, which is used more in Europe than in the US, utilizes a 15 min bath in 10 ml of 1% oxsoralen lotion in 100 L bath water at body temperature followed by UVA exposure. Initial UVA dosing is recommended at 40% of the MPD, with subsequent increases by 20–40% of the initial dose at each treatment. Alternatively bath pUVA may utilize trimethylpsoralen which is administered as 50 mg dissolved in 100 mL of ethanol and mixed in 150 L of water at body temperature. With this, initial UVA therapy is begun at 40% of the MPD and then followed by increases of half of the initial UVA dose at each subsequent visit [122]. Treatment is given two to three times weekly, never on consecutive days.

pUVA soak therapy is used particularly in the treatment of hands and feet. The hands and feet are soaked twice weekly for 15 min in 0.5 ml of 1–2% 8-MOP lotion mixed in 2 liters of water followed by UVA exposure 30 min later. Initial UVA doses are between 1–2 J/cm^2 with incremental increases of 0.5–1 J/cm^2 per treatment. Alternatively, 5 mg of trimethylpsoralen in 10 mL of ethanol can be used, mixed in 15 liters of water [122].

Cream formulations of 8-MOP are generally applied immediately prior to light exposure. Photosensitivity is limited to 2 h post exposure. A small comparative study of pUVA cream and pUVA bath therapy in palmoplantar disease showed similar efficacy between the two modalities [124]. Local application of gel pUVA utilizes a 0.005% solution of aqueous 8-MOP gel, applied thinly over the affected areas 15 min before UVA exposure. Gel pUVA therapy seems to be equivalently effective as bath pUVA [125].

Emollients and ultraviolet A therapy

Very little data exists on the use of emollients in conjunction with UVA phototherapy alone. In a study of various types of emollients used in normal subjects prior to exposure to pUVA, oil-in-water emollients with or without 10% urea significantly reduced the minimal phototoxic dose. This may indicate that such preparations may decrease the total UVA dose required to clear psoriasis [126]. Further clinical studies are required however.

Keratolytics and UVA therapy

Similar to their effects in ultraviolet B therapy, application of salicylic acid immediately prior to UVA phototherapy can increase the minimal phototoxic dose [127]. Thus, although helpful for removing thick scale, salicylic acid should be applied after light treatment, or if used prior to treatment, be washed off completely before phototherapy.

Dithranol and UVA

Few studies have looked at the efficacy of dithranol with UVA since Morison et al. first reported its benefit in 1978. Although anthralin plus pUVA with or without dithranol clears patients' psoriasis more quickly than pUVA does alone, patients tend to dislike the combination regimen, likely secondary to the inconvenience of anthralin [68, 128].

Tar and UVA

Coal tar and pUVA is not used in combination due to increased risk of phototoxicity [129].

Vitamin D derivatives and UVA

Vitamin D derivatives such as calcipotriene cream and ointment have been found to reduce the total dose as well as the duration and number of treatments required to achieve clearance than with pUVA alone [130–134]. Similar results were seen in a trial of tacalcitol and pUVA [135]. The mechanism of action of this combined modality is unknown.

Adverse effects such as irritation and hyperpigmentation have been reported [135, 136]. However, a systematic review of randomized controlled trials of photochemotherapy and topical calcipotriene did not show a difference in the frequency of adverse events in comparison to placebo [59].

Treatment is recommend twice daily with the vitamin D analog in conjunction with three times weekly pUVA therapy [137]. However, because of a known photoprotective effect of calcipotriene when applied just prior to photochemotherapy, and because UVA degrades topical vitamin D derivatives, application is recommended a few hours after phototherapy [138–140].

Tazarotene and UVA

Tzaneva et al. showed that the combination of pUVA plus a thin layer of nightly tazarotene was superior to pUVA alone, with reductions in the cumulative UVA dose and number of exposures needed for clearing. Side effects were minimal and transient and limited to dryness, irritant contact dermatitis, pruritis, and burning sensation. No differences in remission rates were noted [135].

Similarly, tazarotene with bath pUVA resulted in 76% reduction in disease severity compared to 58% with bath pUVA alone after 3 weeks [141]. Thus, like the vitamin D analogs, the addition of tazarotene may play a beneficial role in hastening clearance and in doing so decreases the cumulative associated risks of exposure to pUVA phototherapy.

Corticosteroids and UVA

In contrast to the data on ultraviolet B phototherapy in conjunction with corticosteroids, a literature review by Meola and others of five small studies on the combination of topical steroids with pUVA *versus* pUVA therapy alone showed rapid clearing with smaller cumulative pUVA dosages in patients receiving combined therapy [67]. The combination was also shown to be more beneficial than either modality alone, with rapid normalization of skin and up to 12 weeks of sustained remission [142, 143].

Systemics and UVA

Acitretin and UVA (RepUVA)

Systemic retinoids such as acitretin, isotretinoin, and etretinate, when used in conjunction with photochemotherapy increase pUVA's treatment efficacy while reducing the number, duration, and cumulative doses of pUVA treatments. Tanew et al. showed that 96% of patients cleared with combined therapy with acitretin *versus* 80% with pUVA alone. The cumulative dose to achieve clearance was reduced by 42% and the time to clearance was decreased by over 10 days [144]. Similar results have been demonstrated with other systemic retinoids in combination with systemic or topical pUVA [145–148]. 85% of patients remain relapse free at 6 months with RepUVA [39].

RepUVA therapy can also be effective for those patients with palmoplantar pustulosis. Retinoids cause thinning of the epidermis and stratum corneum, allowing an increased sensitivity to ultraviolet light. Low doses of an oral retinoid in combination with pUVA can result in dramatic improvement in disease while requiring lower overall doses of UVA and avoiding many retinoid associated side effects [149]. Furthermore, retinoids also function to suppress skin cancer formation [150].

Systemic retinoids are usually started 2 weeks prior to commencing photochemotherapy. Given their ability to increase photosensitivity, UVA doses should be lowered by approximately 50% to avoid the risk of burning. Blood monitoring is necessary while patients are on this regimen. Again, care in using systemic retinoids in women of childbearing potential is necessary and their use may be contraindicated as these drugs are potent teratogens.

Methotrexate and UVA

The combination of UVA and methotrexate may be useful for patients with severe psoriasis. In a study by Morison et al., after 3 weeks of methotrexate only, patients were started on four times weekly pUVA in conjunction with the methotrexate. 93% of patients cleared after an average 9.3 pUVA treatments and a mean total dose of 93 milligrams of methotrexate [151]. Like combination therapy with nbUVB, combining methotrexate and pUVA produces more rapid response, requires fewer pUVA treatments and lowers cumulative doses of pUVA and methotrexate [151, 152]. An additive risk of carcinogenesis may exist however with this approach, as both methotrexate and pUVA may independently be associated with an increased risk of skin cancer with long-term use [153]. Additionally, prolonged subacute phototoxicity reactions have been reported [151, 154].

Cyclosporine and UVA

Cyclosporine is known to bring about swift and often long lasting improvement in cases of severe or erythrodermic psoriasis when used in combination with or prior to commencing phototherapy [155, 156]. However, caution is advised as an additive risk of squamous cell skin cancer occurs with the combined use of cyclosporine and ultraviolet A phototherapy. In a cohort of patients who received pUVA, the risk of squamous-cell carcinoma after any use of cyclosporine was three-fold that of those patients who never received cyclosporine. Furthermore, this risk was equal to the independent risk of skin cancer in patients receiving over 200 pUVA treatments in the same cohort [157]. More recently, a second large prospective cohort of psoriatic patients who received cyclosporine reported a 7.3-fold risk of developing non-melanoma skin cancer in patients who also had a history of pUVA [158]. Fortunately, as more options for treatment of severe psoriasis emerge, the need to accept such risks becomes less necessary and long term cyclosporine is therefore considered contraindicated with pUVA.

UVA1

Long wave UVA (340–400 nm) was first described in 1981 and has been used primarily to treat a number of sclerotic and inflammatory disorders. Its use in psoriasis is limited currently to preliminary studies [159]. Ultraviolet A1 radiation induces immediate T-lymphocyte apoptosis through oxidative stress [160]. Various UVA1 light sources are available, which can provide low (10–30 J/cm^2), medium (40–70 J/cm^2), or high (up to 130 J/cm^2) energy outputs. Dosimetry has not been standardized, equipment is not widely available, and for high doses, elaborate cooling systems are necessary [160]. A small nonrandomized comparison of medium dose UVA1 at 50 J/cm^2 *versus* broadband UVB therapy in the same patients showed efficacy of UVA1 in improving psoriatic plaques. However, given the study's small sample size, no difference was detected between UVB and UVA1 phototherapies [161]. Furthermore, in the very small number of psoriatic patients treated thus far in the US, no efficacy has been established [162, 163]. Adverse effects include the possible induction of polymorphous light eruption, erythema, pruritus, tenderness, and burning sensation [162]. In spite of these limitations, the possibility that UVA1 may play a more important role in the treatment of psoriasis in the future exists. Pointing toward this, UVA1 in combination with calcipotriol has been found to be equivalently efficacious to narrowband UVB with calcipotriol therapy and more efficacious than calcipotriol alone in a randomized controlled trial [164].

Narrowband UVB *versus* pUVA

Narrowband UVB therapy and pUVA have clearly demonstrated efficacy in the treatment of psoriasis. However, narrowband UVB therapy has become more frequently utilized because it offers greater relative safety and convenience in comparison to pUVA. It also can be used more safely in women should they become pregnant, and in children. It is considered safer for skin type I or those with a history of radiation or arsenic treatment as these patients are at higher risk for development of skin cancer with pUVA. Narrowband UVB is preferred over pUVA for patients with recent initial onset of disease or for younger patients in order to minimize cumulative UV exposures. However, pUVA penetrates more deeply into the skin than UVB and is more effective. Thus pUVA has an advantage for thicker plaques, palm or sole involvement or for aggressive disease, e.g., erythrodermic or pustular psoriasis. Furthermore, pUVA also offers the advantage of longer induced remissions than with UVB [6].

Combination UVA and UVB

The combination of concurrent UVA alone and UVB phototherapy is used rarely, although pUVA and UVB have been successfully used concurrently. A small intrapatient controlled study of eight patients given UVB only or combination UVA and UVB failed to show a difference in efficacy [165]. On the other hand, combination therapy utilizing broadband UVB and systemic pUVA three times weekly did produce clearing more rapidly and with lower respective cumulative UVA and UVB doses than with either modality alone [166]. Additionally, topical bath and cream pUVA targeted treatment of plaques in patients undergoing narrowband UVB phototherapy have shown similar results [167, 168]. However, concern exists regarding increased phototoxicity with the use of narrowband light in patients being treated with bath pUVA [167]. Treatment is generally indicated for patients who fail individual therapy or who flare on home UVB. pUVA can be given twice weekly in addition to the patient's regular home UVB regimen, with phototherapy sessions separated by 24 h to ensure psoralen blood levels are zero before exposure to UVB. For the most part this combination has become less utilized given the increased number of systemic alternatives.

Commercial tanning beds

Some patients, for whom office-based phototherapy is not feasible, with or without the advice of their physicians, obtain treatment with commercial tanning beds. Commercial tanning lamps generally have outputs in the UVA range. However, a fraction of the emission, anywhere from less than 1–9% can be in the UVB range, depending on the pressure and age of the bulbs. Although studies using commercial lamps emitting less than 1% UVB have shown improvement in psoriasis, greater efficacy is achieved with lamps having a higher overall percentage of output in the UVB spectrum. Thus patient convenience of attending a local salon must be weighed against the inherent inconsistencies of dosing, the limited exposure to UVB, the difficulty of achieving efficacious UVA dosing, the lack of medical supervision, and the medicolegal liability associated with this modality [169].

Other combinations

Hydroxyurea

There is limited information about the use of hydroxyurea in combination with either UVB phototherapy or pUVA [68, 170]. Oral dosing of 500 mg twice daily is recommended in conjunction with light treatment. Its use is recommended for patients who respond incompletely to UVB alone, who may be averse to liver biopsy or who have cirrhosis. Although it does not seem to carry an increased risk of photosensitivity and has a minimal risk of hepatotoxicity, its narrow therapeutic index behooves a cautious approach, with CBC, LFT, and renal function monitoring recommended [171]. Finally, hydroxyurea is teratogenic and therefore contraindicated in pregnancy.

Biologics

Recent studies looking at combination therapy of ultraviolet light and the new biologics have promising results. In an open label trial comparing alefacept monotherapy with alefacept in combination with either narrowband or with broadband ultraviolet light, higher overall response rates and more rapid onset of responses were noted with in both combined treatment arms than with either types of light therapy alone or alefacept alone. There was no evidence for increased rate of phototoxicity or photosensitivity. However, no measures of statistical significance were reported [172]. Furthermore, case reports of patients with therapy-resistant psoriasis achieving complete clearance after receiving alefacept followed by narrowband UVB have begun to emerge [173].

Another one of the new targeted biologic agents, efalizumab, is currently being studied as part of a 36 month continuous therapy regimen in which 6% of the enrolled patients are on concurrent ultraviolet B phototherapy. Although data on the patients receiving concomitant therapies or phototherapy in particular is not separately reported, thus far the efficacy and safety data seem to indicate that efalizumab may be successfully used in combination with other psoriasis treatment modalities [174]. Furthermore, a report of five patients treated with etanercept and narrowband UVB points toward increased efficacy, and decreased onset of action, without increased side effects using the combined modalities [175]. No studies thus far have been reported in this area with ultraviolet A. In general, as the current biologic therapies are known to be immunosuppressive, it remains to be seen whether there is a long-term increased risk of skin malignancy with combination use with light treatments.

Phototherapy in special populations

Elderly

Phototherapy may be a useful option in those patients with comorbidities or concomitant medications that interact with topical or systemic agents used to treat psoriasis, e.g., hypertension, renal impairment, poor eyesight, neurological impairment, or physical disability. However, many elderly patients are on photosensitizing drugs, may not tolerate prolonged standing, or may not be able to travel to the phototherapy center. Eligible elderly patients include those who are ambulatory, can attend sessions at least three times weekly, can tolerate standing for up to 15 min at a time, do not have cataracts, are not on photosensitizing medications, and do not have a history of skin cancer or risk factors for development of skin cancer (arsenic or radiation exposure). Phototherapy units serving the elderly need to be equipped with non slip mats, railings, steps and emergency call bells. Moisturization should be aggressive as phototherapy may initially aggravate xerosis and pruritis, conditions which are already common in this patient population [176].

Children

Although few studies have been done on ultraviolet B therapy in children with psoriasis, UVB is considered relatively safe and effective in this population. In a retrospective review of 77 patients less than 16 years of age who received nbUVB over 7 years, 63% of children being treated with psoriasis had minimal residual disease after a median of 17.5 treatments. In comparison to adults treated at the same centers, narrowband therapy is less effective in children, with 89% of psoriatic adults achieving minimal residual disease. The authors of this study offer a selection-bias hypothesis for this discrepancy; given the limited data in children and concerns for side effects, only children with severe disease are selected for treatment whereas narrowband therapy in adults is used for mild to moderate disease [177]. Similar response rates in children have been noted by other studies [178]. The adverse effect profile was similar in children as it is in adults: erythema, blistering, PMLE, and HSV reactivation were all noted, although a percent breakdown of these adverse events occurring specifically in children treated for psoriasis was not noted. Anxiety was an additional reported problem in a small number of the patients [177]. No studies exist on the long-term risk of carcinogenesis in children who have received ultraviolet B light. Its use is limited, therefore, to second line therapy in those children whose disease fails topical treatments.

In general, given the known increased risk of cancer with pUVA in adults, pUVA treatment in children less than 10 years old is reserved for exceptional cases in which all other more optimal treatments have failed and the risk-benefit ratio justifies the treatment. In a series of 26 patients younger than 16 who received pUVA treatment, one patient developed two basal cell cancers before age 21. This patient was one of five children in the group who received greater than 200 treatments [179]. Because of their greater body surface to body mass ratios, children who do receive pUVA treatment, either orally or topically, must wear eye protection. This is in contrast to adults, who do not require eye protection with topical psoralen application [180]. Bath therapy is preferred over systemic therapy because it produces less nausea and has a shorter duration of photosensitization [181]. Unfortunately, bath phototherapy is not available in the United States. Like adults, genital shielding is essential.

Additionally, parents should be counseled regarding the increased risk of photoaging with the use of photochemotherapy and UVB light treatments and methods to minimize ambient childhood sun exposures should be discussed. Combination approaches with topicals and phototherapy are recommended to optimize therapeutic response and thus minimize ultraviolet exposure as much as possible. Also, attempts should also be made to make the phototherapy environment as child-friendly as possible to reduce the impact of anxiety. Finally, parents of small children unable to stand on their own or afraid of closed spaces may need to enter the phototherapy booth, wearing complete photoprotective clothing, with their child during treatments.

Pregnancy

Although 30–65% of women experience some improvement in their psoriasis during pregnancy, some whose psoriasis is unable to be controlled with topical agents will require more aggressive treatment. Some systemic modalities, including acitretin and methotrexate are contraindicated in pregnancy, whereas others such as cyclosporine are considered options in selected cases only. Thus, phototherapy may play a more prominent role in the treatment of these patients. UVB is preferred for extensive psoriasis [182]. Systemic pUVA has not been associated with increased rates of teratogenicity [183]. Although teratogenicity has not been studied, topical or bath treatment is preferable to oral photochemotherapy in those patients whose psoriasis requires pUVA, in order to limit exposure to psoralen [184].

Future developments in light therapy

Bexarotene

Bexarotene, a novel retinoid targeting the retinoid-X receptor has been used in the treatment of cutaneous T-cell lymphomas for its apoptotic and antiproliferative properties. In the past half-decade, recent studies on its application in psoriasis have begun emerging. Systemic administration of bexarotene alone has demonstrated improvement in proliferation, differentiation and inflammation in psoriatic plaques [185]. The same study group also found systemic treatment to have clinical efficacy with adverse effects limited to hypertriglyceridemia and central hypothyroidism [186]. Furthermore, in a subset of these patients, combining systemic bexarotene administration with ultraviolet B light did not have any effect on the minimal erythema dose nor did it cause photosensitivity after one dose [187]. A separate group recently published a pilot study of bexarotene gel in combination with narrowband therapy. Significant improvement in induration of target lesions was noted over narrowband therapy alone. Side effects were similar to those of other topical retinoids and limited to erythema, pain and pruritis [188]. Thus, although utilization of this novel RXR specific retinoid in psoriasis is still in its early stages, results thus far promise the possibility of successful combination treatments with light therapy.

Photodynamic therapy

Reports of off-label use of systemic and topical photodynamic therapy (PDT), utilizing a photosensitizer such as a porphyrin, for the treatment of psoriasis have recently begun emerging in the literature. Administration of topical and systemic aminolevulinic acid (ALA) induces selective accumulation of protoporphyrin IX (pPIX) in psoriatic plaques. Blue light exposure of ALA treated skin results in photobleaching, with erythema and reduction in pPIX fluorescence. Proposed mechanisms of action for efficacy of PDT in psoriasis include dose dependent inhibition of TNF alpha, ILF-1, and IL-6 secretions, similar to the effects seen in pUVA therapy. Additionally, apoptosis of CD3 cells has been noted with systemic aminolevulinic acid (ALA). PDT has also been shown to decrease epidermal proliferation, normalize epidermal differentiation, reduce epidermal CD8 T cells and diminish epidermal and dermal memory T cells in psoriasis [189].

Efficacy of photodynamic therapy in comparison to established treatment modalities such as narrowband UVB for psoriasis is questionable [190]. ALA is the photosensitizer most commonly used. A number of different types of light sources have been utilized including diode lasers and visible light projectors [191]. No uniform treatment protocol has yet been established and inconsistencies in accumulation of the photosensitizer, in protoporphyrin IX fluorescence after ALA application, and most importantly, in patient response have been reported [192]. Additionally, koebnerization and severe patient discomfort during the treatment remain limiting adverse effects of this modality. Furthermore, long-term safety remains to be established. No large scale trials exist at this time.

Conclusion

Phototherapy and photochemotherapy in their various forms have proven efficacy for the treatment of psoriasis. Major advantages of these modalities include the ability to treat multiple body sites and usefulness in patients of all ages. Limitations exist however in accessibility to treatment centers and the potential risk of skin cancer. Exciting new developments in this field of treatment continue to emerge.

References

1 Lebwohl M, Ting PT, Koo JY (2005) Psoriasis treatment: traditional therapy. *Ann Rheum Dis* 64S2: ii83–86
2 Ingram JT (1953) The approach to psoriasis. *Br J Dermatol* 2: 591–594
3 Stuttgen G (1997) History of treatments. *Clin Dermatol* 15: 693–703
4 Zanolli M (2004) Phototherapy arsenal in the treatment of psoriasis. *Dermatol Clin* 22: 397–406
5 Green C, Diffey BL, Hawk JL (1992) Ultraviolet radiation in the treatment of skin disease. *Physics Med Biol* 37(1): 1–20
6 Naldi L, Griffiths CEM (2005) Traditional therapies in the management of moderate to severe chronic plaque psoriasis: an assessment of the benefits and risks. *B J Dermatol* 152 (4): 597–615
7 Bonis B, Kemeny L, Dobozy A, Bor Z, Szabo G, Ignacz F (1997) 308 nm UVB excimer laser for psoriasis. *Lancet* 350(9090): 1522
8 Hacker SM, Rasmussen JE (1992) The effect of flash lamp-pulsed dye laser on psoriasis. *Arch Dermatol* 128: 853–855

9 Al-Ajmi HS (2006) A comparison of minimal erythema doses for narrowband *versus* broadband ultraviolet B irradiation in darkly pigmented healthy subjects and in psoriatic patients in Kuwait. *Br J Dermatol* 154: 774–807
10 Lebwohl M (2000) Advances in psoriasis therapy. *Dermatol Clin* 18(1): 13–9, vii
11 Coven TR, Burack LH, Gilleaudeau P, Keogh M, Ozawa M, Kreuger JG (1997) Narrowband UV-B produces superior clinical and histopathological resolution of moderate-to-severe-psoriasis in patients compared with broadband UV-B. *Arch Dermatol* 133(12): 1514–1522
12 Dawe RS (2003) A quantitative review of studies comparing the efficacy of narrow-band and broad-band ultraviolet B for psoriasis. *Br J Dermatol* 149: 669–672
13 Berneburg M, Rocken M, Benedix F (2005) Phototherapy with narrowband *versus* broadband UVB. *Acta Derm Venereol* 85(2): 98–108
14 Bandow GD, Koo JYM (2004) Narrow-band ultraviolet B radiation: a review of the current literature. *Int J Dermatol* 43: 555–561
15 Weishcer M, Blum A, Eberhard F, Rocken M, Berneburg M (2004) No evidence for increased skin cancer risk in psoriasis patients treated with broadband or narrowband UVB photo therapy: a first retrospective study. *Acta Derm Venereol* 84: 370–374
16 Man I, Crombie IK, Dawe RS, Ibbotson SH, Ferguson J (2005) The photocarcinogenic risk of narrowband UVB (TL-01) phototherapy: early follow-up data. *Br J Dermatol* 152: 755–757
17 Lee E, Koo J, Berger T (2005) UVB phototherapy and skin cancer risk: a review of the literature. *Int J Dermatol* 44(5): 355–360
18 Ibbotson SH, Bilsland D, Cox NH, Dawe RS, Diffey B, Edwards C, Farr PM, Ferguson J, Hart G, Hawk J (2004) An update and guidance on narrowband ultraviolet B photo therapy: a British Photodermatology Group Workshop Report. *Br J Dermatol* 151: 283–297
19 Green C, Ferguson J, Lakshmipathi T, Johnson BE (1988) 311 nm UVB phototherapy – an effective treatment for psoriasis. *Br J Dermatol* 119(6): 691–696
20 Kenicer KJA, Lakshmipathi T, Addo HA (1981) An assessment of the effect of photochemotherapy (PUVA) and UVB phototherapy in the treatment of psoriasis. *Br J Dermatol* 105: 629–639
21 Eells LD, Wolff JM, Garloff J, Eaglstein WH (1984) Comparison of suberythemogenic and maximally aggressive ultraviolet B therapy for psoriasis. *J Am Acad Dermatol* 11(1): 105–110
22 Cameron H, Dawe RS, Yule S, Murphy J, Ibbotson SH, Ferguson J (2002) A randomized, observer-blinded trial of twice *versus* three times weekly narrowband ultraviolet B phototherapy for chronic plaque psoriasis. *Br J Dermatol* 147(5): 973–978
23 Dawe RS, Wainwright NJ, Cameron H, Ferguson J (1998) Narrowband (TL-01) ultraviolet B phototherapy for chronic plaque psoriasis: three times or five times weekly treatment? *Br J Dermatol* 138: 833–839
24 Leenutaphong V, Nimkulrat P, Sudtim S (2000) Comparison of phototherapy two times and four times a week with low doses of narrow-band ultraviolet B in Asian patients with psoriasis. *Photodermatol Photoimmunol Photomed* 16: 202–206
25 Otman SG, Edwards C, Pearse AD, Gambles BJ, Anstey AV (2006) Modulation of ultraviolet (UV) transmission by emollients: relevance to narrowband UVB phototherapy and psoralen plus UVA photochemotherapy. *Br J Dermatol* 154(5): 963–968
26 Berne B, Blom I, Spangberg S (1990) Enhanced response of psoriasis to UVB therapy after pretreatment with a lubricating base. A single-blind controlled study. *Acta Dermato-Venereologica* 70(6): 474–477
27 Penven K, Leroy D, Verneuil L, Faguer K, Dompmartin A (2005) Evaluation of vaseline oil applied prior to UVB TL01 phototherapy in the treatment of psoriasis. *Photodermatol Photoimmunol Photomed* 21(3): 138–141
28 Fetil E, Ozka S, Soyal MC, Ilknur T, Erdem Y, Gunes AT (2002) Effects of topical petrolatum and salicylic acid on the erythemogenicity of UVB. *Eur J Dermatol* 12: 154–156
29 Lebwohl M, Martinez J, Weber P, DeLuca R (1995) Effects of topical preparations on the erythemogenicity of UVB: implications for psoriasis phototherapy. *J Am Acad Dermatol* 32(3): 469–471
30 Kristensen B, Kristensen O (1991) Topical salicylic acid interferes with UVB therapy for psoriasis. *Acta Derm Venereol* 71(1): 37–40
31 Harber LC, Armstrong RB, Leach EE (1981) Preliminary report: Modified Goeckerman therapy for hospitalized patients: Ambulatory day care center and improved quantitative dosimetry. *J Invest Dermatol* 77: 162–166
32 Armstrong RB, Leach EE, Fleiss JL, Harber LC (1984) Modified Goeckerman therapy for psori-

asis. A two-year follow-up of a combined hospital-ambulatory care program. *Arch Dermatol* 120: 313–318
33 Lee E, Koo J (2005) Modern modified 'ultra' Goeckerman therapy: a PASI assessment of a very effective therapy for psoriasis resistant to both prebiologic and biologic therapies. *J Dermatol Treat* 16: 102–107
34 Marsico AR, Eaglstein WH, Weinstein GD (1976) Ultraviolet light and tar in the Goeckerman treatment of psoriasis. *Arch Dermatol* 112: 1249–1250
35 Petrozzi JW, Barton JO, Kaidbey KK, Kligman AM (1978) Updating the Goeckerman regimen for psoriasis. *Br J Dermatol* 98: 437–444
36 Lowe NJ, Wortzman MS, Breeding J, Koudsi H, Taylor L (1983) Coal tar phototherapy for psoriasis reevaluated: erythemogenic *versus* suberythemogenic ultraviolet with a tar extract in oil and crude coal tar. *J Am Acad Dermatol* 8: 781–789
37 Dodd WA (1993) Tars. Their role in the treatment of psoriasis. *Dermatol Clin* 11(1): 131–135
38 Menter A, Cram DL (1983) The Goeckerman regimen in two psoriasis day care centers. *J Am Acad Dermatol* 9: 59–65
39 Koo J, Lebwohl M (1999) Duration of remission of psoriasis therapies. *J Am Acad Dermatol* 41: 51–59
40 Borska L, Fiala Z, Smejkalova J, Hamakova K, Kremlacek J (2004) Possible genotoxic risk of combined exposure to pharmaceutical coal tar and UV-B radiation. *Central Eur J Public Health* 12: S14–15
41 Pion IA, Koenig KL, Lim HW (1995) Is dermatologic usage of coal tar carcinogenic? A review of the literature. *Dermatol Surg* 21: 227–231
42 Pittelkow MR, Perry HO, Muller SA, Maughan WZ, O'Brien PC (1981) Skin cancer in patients with psoriasis treated with coal tar: a 25 year follow-up study. *Arch Dermatol* 117: 465–468
43 Ryatt KS, Statham BN, Rowell NR (1984) Short-contact modification of the Ingram regime. *Br J Dermatol* 111(4): 455–459
44 McBride SR, Walker P, Reynolds NJ (2003) Optimizing the frequency of outpatient short-contact dithranol treatment used in combination with broadband ultraviolet B for psoriasis: a randomized, within-patient controlled trial. *Br J Dermatol* 149: 1259–1265
45 Karvonen J, Kokkonen EL, Ruotsalainen E (1989) 311 nm UVB lamps in the treatment of psoriasis with the Ingram regimen. *Acta Derm Venereol* 69(1): 82–85
46 Seville RH (1975) Simplified dithranol treatment for psoriasis. *Br J Dermatol* 93: 205–208
47 Statham BN, Ryatt KS, Rowell NR (1984) Short-contact dithranol therapy – a comparison with the Ingram regime. *Br J Dermatol* 110: 703–708
48 Paramsothy Y, Collins M, Lawrence CM (1988) Effect of UVB therapy and a coal tar bath on short contact dithranol treatment for psoriasis. *Br J Dermatol* 118: 783–789
49 Behrens S, Grundmann-Kollman M, Schiener R, Peter RU, Kerscher M (2000) Combination phototherapy of psoriasis with narrow-band UVB irradiation and topical tazarotene gel. *J Am Acad Dermatol* 42: 493–495
50 van de Kerkhof PCM (2006) Update on retinoid therapy of psoriasis in: an update on the use of retinoids in dermatology. *Dermatol Ther* 19(5): 252–263
51 Takahashi H, Ibe M, Kinouchi M, Ishida-Yamamoto A, Hashimoto Y, Iizuka H (2003) Similarly potent action of 1,25-dihydroxyvitamin D3 and its analogues, tacalcitol, calcipotriol, and maxacalcitol on normal human keratinocyte proliferation and differentiation. *J Dermatol Sci* 31(1): 21–28
52 Berneburg M, Röcken M, Benedix F (2005) Phototherapy with Narrowband *versus* Broadband UVB. Phototherapy with Narrowband *versus* Broadband UVB. *Acta Derm Venereol* 85: 98–108
53 Roussaki-Schulze AV, Kouskoukis C, Klimi E, Zafiriou E, Galanos A, Rallis E (2005) Calcipotriol monotherapy *versus* calcipotriol plus UVA1 *versus* calcipotriol plus narrow-band UVB in the treatment of psoriasis. *Drugs Exper Clin Res* 31(5–6): 169–174
54 Brazzelli V, Barbagallo T, Prestinari F, Rona C, De Silvestri A, Trevisan V, Borroni G (2005) Non-invasive evaluation of tacalcitol plus puva *versus* tacalcitol plus UVB-NB in the treatment of psoriasis: "right-left intra-individual pre/post comparison design". *Int J Immunopath Pharm* 18(4): 755–760
55 Molin L (1999) Topical calcipotriol combined with phototherapy for psoriasis. The results of two randomized trials and a review of the literature. Calcipotriol-UVB Study Group. *Dermatology* 198(4): 375–381
56 Messer G, Degitz K, Plewig G, Rocken M (2001) Pretreatment of psoriasis with the vitamin D3

derivative tacalcitol increases the responsiveness to 311-nm ultraviolet B: results of a controlled, right/left study. Pretreatment of psoriasis with the vitamin D3 derivative tacalcitol increases the responsiveness to 311-nm ultraviolet B: results of a controlled, right/left study. *Br J Dermatol* 144(3): 628–629

57 Rim JH, Choe YB, Youn JI (2002) Positive effect of using calcipotriol ointment with narrow-band ultraviolet B phototherapy in psoriatic patients. *Photodermatol Photoimmunol Photomed* 18: 131–134

58 Ring J, Kowalzick L, Christophers E, Schill WB, Schopf E, Stander M, Wolff HH, Altmeyer P (2001) Calcitriol 3 microg g-1 ointment in combination with ultraviolet B phototherapy for the treatment of plaque psoriasis: results of a comparative study. *Br J Dermatol* 144: 495–499

59 Ashcroft DM, Li Wan Po A, Williams HC, Griffiths CE (2000) Combination regimens of topical calcipotriene in chronic plaque psoriasis: systematic review of efficacy and tolerability. *Arch Dermatol* 136(12): 1536–1543

60 Woo WK, McKenna KE (2003) Combination TL01 ultraviolet B phototherapy and topical calcipotriol for psoriasis: a prospective randomized placebo-controlled clinical trial. *Br J Dermatol* 149(1): 146–150

61 de Rie MA, de Hoop D, Jonsson L, Bakkers EJ, Sorensen M (2001) Pharmacoeconomic evaluation of calcipotriol (Daivonex/Dovonex) and UVB phototherapy in the treatment of psoriasis: a Markov model for The Netherlands. *Dermatol* 202(1): 38–43

62 Ramsay CA, Schwartz BE, Lowson D, Papp K, Bolduc A, Gilbert M (2000) Calcipotriol cream combined with twice weekly broad-band UVB phototherapy: a safe, effective and UVB-sparing antipsoriatric combination treatment. The Canadian Calcipotriol and UVB Study Group. *Dermatol* 200(1): 17–24

63 Molin L (1999) Topical calcipotriol combined with phototherapy for psoriasis. The results of two randomized trials and a review of the literature. Calcipotriol-UVB Study Group. *Dermatol* 198(4): 375–381

64 Lebwohl M, Quijije J, Gilliard J, Rollin T, Watts O (2003) Topical calcitriol is degraded by ultraviolet light. *J Invest Dermatol* 121(3): 594–595

65 Lebwohl M, Hecker D, Martinez J, Sapadin A, Patel B (1997) Interactions between calcipotriene and ultraviolet light. *J Am Acad Dermatol* 37(1): 93–95

66 McKenna KE, Stern RS (1995) Photosensitivity associated with combined UV-B and calcipotriene therapy. *Arch Dermatol* 131(11): 1305–1307

67 Meola T, Soter NA, Lim HW (1991) Are topical corticosteroids useful adjunctive therapy for the treatment of psoriasis with ultraviolet radiation? A review of the literature. *Arch Dermatol* 127(11): 1708–1713

68 Lebwohl M, Menter A, Koo J, Feldman SR (2004) Combination therapy to treat moderate to severe psoriasis. *J Am Acad Dermatol* 50(3): 416–430

69 Matz H, Orion E, Wolf R (2003) Balneotherapy in dermatology. *Dermatol Ther* 16(2): 132–140

70 Hodak E, Gottlieb AB, Segal T, Politi Y, Maron L, Sulkes J, David M (2003) Climatotherapy at the Dead Sea is a remittive therapy for psoriasis: combined effects on epidermal and immunologic activation. *J Am Acad Dermatol* 49(3): 451–457

71 Tsoureli-Nikita E, Menchini G, Ghersetich I, Hercogova J (2002) Alternative treatment of psoriasis with balneotherapy using Leopoldine spa water. J Eur Acad Dermatol Venereol 16(3): 260–262

72 Holló P, Gonzalez R, Kása M, Horváth A (2005) Synchronous balneophototherapy is effective for the different clinical types of psoriasis. *J Eur Acad Dermatol Venereol* 19(5): 578–581

73 Léauté-Labrèze C, Saillour F, Chene G, Cazenave C, Luxey-Bellocq ML, Sanciaume C, Toussaint JF, Taieb A (2001) Saline spa water or combined water and UV-B for psoriasis *versus* conventional UV-B: lessons from the Salies de Béarn randomized study. *Arch Dermatol* 137: 1035–1039

74 Harari M, Shani J (1997) Demographic evaluation of successful antipsoriatic climatotherapy at the Dead Sea (Israel) DMZ clinic. *Int J Dermatol* 36: 304–308

75 David M, Efron D, Hodak E, Even-Paz Z (2000) Treatment of psoriasis at the Dead Sea: Why, how and when? *IMAJ* 2: 232–234

76 Dawe RS, Yule S, Cameron H, Moseley H, Ibbotson SH, Ferguson J (2005) A randomized controlled comparison of the efficacy of Dead Sea salt balneophototherapy *versus* narrowband ultraviolet B monotherapy for chronic plaque psoriasis. *Br J Dermatol* 153(3): 613–619

77 Larko O, Swanbeck G (1979) Home solarium treatment of psoriasis. *B J Dermatol* 101: 13–16

78 Cameron H, Yule S, Moseley H, Dawe RS, Ferguson J (2002) Taking treatment to the patient: development of a home TL-01 ultraviolet B phototherapy service. *Br J Dermatol* 147: 957–965

79 Yelverton CB, Kulkarni AS, Balkrishnan R, Feldman SR (2006) Home ultraviolet B phototherapy: a cost-effective option for severe psoriasis. *Managed Care Interface* 19(1): 33–36, 39
80 Koek MBG, Buskens E, Bruijnzeel-Koomen CAFM, Sigurdsson V (2006) Home ultraviolet B phototherapy for psoriasis: discrepancy between literature, guidelines, general opinions and actual use. Results of a literature review, a web search, and a questionnaire among dermatologists. *B J Dermatol* 154: 701–711
81 Sarkany RPE, Anstey A, Diffey BL, Jobling R, Langmack K, McGregor JM, Moseley H, Murphy GM, Rhodes LE, Norris PG; British Photodermatology Group (1999) Home phototherapy: report on a workshop of the British Photodermatology Group, December 1996. *Br J Dermatol* 140: 195–199
82 Ruzicka T, Sommerburg C, Braun-Falco O, Koster W, Lengen W, Lensing W, Letzel H, Meigel WN, Paul E, Przybilla B et al. (1990) Efficiency of acitretin in combination with UV-B in the treatment of severe psoriasis. *Arch Dermatol* 126: 482–486
83 Iest J, Boer J (1989) Combined treatment of psoriasis with acitretin and UVB phototherapy compared with acitretin alone and UVB alone. *Br J Dermatol* 120: 665–670
84 Lowe NJ, Prystowsky JH, Bourget T, Edelstein J, Nychay S, Armstrong R (1991) Acitretin plus UVB therapy for psoriasis. Comparisons with placebo plus UVB and acitretin alone. *J Am Acad Dermatol* 24(4): 591–594
85 Spuls PI, Rozenblit M, Lebwohl M (2003) Retrospective study of the efficacy of narrowband UVB and acitretin. *J Dermatol Treat* 14(S2): 17–20
86 Green C, Lakshmipathi T, Johnson BE, Ferguson JA (1992) Comparison of the efficacy and relapse rates of narrowband UVB (TL-01) monotherapy *versus* etretinate (re-TL-01) *versus* etretinate-PUVA (re-PUVA) in the treatment of psoriasis patients. *Br J Dermatol* 127: 5–9
87 Kopp T, Karlhofer F, Szepfalusi Z, Schneeberger A, Stingl G, Tanew A (2004) Successful use of acitretin in conjunction with narrowband ultraviolet B phototherapy in a child with severe pustular psoriasis, von Zumbusch type. *Br J Dermatol* 151: 912–916
88 Asawanonda P, Nateetongrungsak Y (2006) Methotrexate plus narrowband UVB phototherapy *versus* narrowband UVB phototherapy alone in the treatment of plaque-type psoriasis: a randomized, placebo-controlled study. *J Am Acad Dermatol* 54(6): 1013–1018
89 Paul BS, Momtaz K, Stern RS, Arndt KA, Parrish JA (1982) Combined methotrexate-ultraviolet B therapy in the treatment of psoriasis. *J Am Acad Dermatol* 7(6): 758–762
90 de Berker DA, Sakuntabhai A, Diffey BL, Matthews JN, Farr PM (1997) Comparison of psoralen-UVB and psoralen-UVA photochemotherapy in the treatment of psoriasis. *J Am Acad Dermatol* 36: 5775–5781
91 Shamsuddin S, Haroon TS (2003) Comparative study of psoralen-UVB *versus* UVB-alone therapy in the treatment of psoriasis. *J Pak Assoc Dermatol* 13: 55–61
92 Ortel B, Perl S, Kinaciyan T, Calzavara-Pinton PG, Hönigsmann H (1993) Comparison of narrow-band (311 nm) UVB and broad-band UVA after oral or bath-water 8-methoxypsoralen in the treatment of psoriasis, *J Am Acad Dermatol* 29: 736–740
93 Amornpinyokeit N, Asawanonda P (2006) 8-methoxypsoralen cream plus targeted narrowband ultraviolet B for psoriasis. *Photodermatol Photoimmunol Photomed* 22: 285–289
94 Bianchi B, Campolmi P, Mavilia L, Danesi A, Rossi R, Cappugi P (2003) Monochromatic excimer light (308 nm): an immunohistochemical study of cutaneous T cells and apoptosis-related molecules in psoriasis. *J Eur Acad Dermatol Venerol* 17: 408–413
95 Novák Z, Bónis B, Baltás E, Ocsovszki I, Ignácz F, Dobozy A, Kemény L (2002) Xenon chloride ultraviolet B laser is more effective in treating psoriasis and in inducing T cell apoptosis than narrow-band ultraviolet B. *J Photochem Photobiol* 67: 32–38
96 Taibjee SM, Cheung ST, Laube S, Lanigan SW (2005) Controlled study of excimer and pulsed dye lasers in the treatment of psoriasis. *Br J Dermatol* 153(5): 960–966
97 Bonis B, Kemeny L, Dobozy A, Bor Z, Szabo G, Ignacz F (1997) 308 nm UVB excimer laser for psoriasis. *Lancet* 350: 1522
98 Gerber W, Arheilger B, Ha TA, Hermann J, Ockenfels HM (2003) Ultraviolet B 308-nm excimer laser treatment of psoriasis: a new phototherapeutic approach. *Br J Dermatol* 149: 1250–1258
99 Mafong EA, Friedman PM, Kauvar AN, Bernstein LJ, Alexiades-Armenakas M, Geronemus RG (2002) Treatment of inverse psoriasis with the 308 nm excimer laser. *Dermatol Surg* 28(6): 530–532
100 Taylor CR, Racette AL (2004) A 308-nm excimer laser for the treatment of scalp psoriasis. *Laser Surg Med* 34(2): 136–140

101 Neumann NJ, Mahnke N, Korpusik D, Stege H, Ruzicka T (2006) Treatment of palmoplantar psoriasis with monochromatic excimer light (308-nm) *versus* cream PUVA. *Acta Derm Venereol* 86: 22–24
102 Acland KM, Barlow BJ (2000) Lasers for the dermatologist. *B J Dermatol* 143: 244–255
103 Zelickson BD, Mehregan DA, Wendelschfer-Crabb G, Ruppman D, Cook A, O'Connell P, Kennedy WR (1996) Clinical and histologic evaluation of psoriatic plaques treated with a flash-lamp pulsed dye laser. *J Am Acad Dermatol* 35: 64–68
104 Hern S, Allen MH, Sousa AR, Harland CC, Barker JNWN, Levick JR, Mortimer PS (2001) Immunohistochemical evaluation of psoriatic plaques following selective photothermolysis of the superficial capillaries. *Br J Dermatol* 145: 45–53
105 de Leeuw J, Tank B, Bjerring PJ, Koetsveld S, Neumann M (2006) Concomitant treatment of psoriasis of the hands and feet with pulsed dye laser and topical calcipotriol, salicylic acid, or both: a prospective open study in 41 patients. *J Am Acad Dermatol* 54(2): 266–271
106 Erceg A, Bovenschen HJ, van de Kerkhof PCM, Seyger MMB (2006) Efficacy of the pulsed dye laser in the treatment of localized recalcitrant plaque psoriasis: a comparative study. *B J Dermatol* 155: 110–114
107 Su J, Pearce DJ, Feldman SR (2005) The role of commercial tanning beds and ultraviolet A light in the treatment of psoriasis. *J Dermatol Treatment* 16(5/6): 324–326
108 Turner RJ, Walshaw D, Diffey BL, Farr PM (2000) A controlled study of ultraviolet A sunbed treatment of psoriasis. *Br J Dermatol* 143: 957–963
109 Coven TR, Walters IB, Cardinale I, Krueger JG (1999) PUVA-induced lymphocyte apoptosis: mechanism of action in psoriasis. *Photodermatol Photoimmunol Photomed* 15: 22–27
110 Tanew A, Ortel B, Honigsmann H (1999) Half-side comparison of erythemogenic *versus* suberythemogenic UVA doses in oral photochemotherapy of psoriasis. *J Am Acad Dermatol* 41(3 Pt 1): 408–413
111 Methoxsalen: drug information. 1978–2006 Lexi-Comp, Inc
112 Stern RS, Lunder EJ (1998) Risk of squamous cell carcinoma and methoxsalen (psoralen) and UV-A radiation (PUVA). A meta-analysis. *Arch Dermatol* 134: 1582–1585
113 Stern RS, Bagheri S, Nichols K (2002) The persistent risk of genital tumors among men treated with psoralen plus ultraviolet A (PUVA) for psoriasis. *J Am Acad Dermatol* 47: 33
114 Stern RS (1999) Genital tumors among men with psoriasis exposed to psoralens and ultraviolet A radiation (PUVA) and ultraviolet B radiation. The Photochemotherapy Follow-up Study. *N Eng J Med* 322(16): 1093–1097
115 Stern RS and PUVA followup study (2001) The risk of melanoma in association with long-term exposure to PUVA. *J Am Acad Dermatol* 44: 755–761
116 Morison WL, Baughman RD, Day RM, Forbes PD, Hoenigsmann H, Krueger GG, Lebwohl M, Lew R, Naldi L, Parrish JA et al. (1998) Consensus workshop on the toxic effects of long-term PUVA therapy. *Arch Dermatol* 134(5): 595–598
117 Hannuksela-Svahn A, Sigurgeirsson B, Pukkala E, Lindelof B, Berne B, Hannuksela M, Poikolainen K, Karvonen J (1999) Trioxsalen bath PUVA did not increase the risk of squamous cell skin carcinoma and cutaneous malignant melanoma in a joint analysis of 944 Swedish and Finnish patients with psoriasis. *Br J Dermatol* 141(3): 497–501
118 Hannuksela-Svahn A, Pukkala E, Koulu L, Jansen CT, Karvonen J (1999) Cancer incidence among Finnish psoriasis patients treated with 8-methoxypsoralen bath PUVA. *J Am Acad Dermatol* 40(5 Pt 1): 694–696
119 Lindelof B, Sigurgeirsson B, Tegner E, Larko O, Johannesson A, Berne B, Ljunggren B, Andersson T, Molin L, Nylander-Lundqvist E et al. (1999) PUVA and cancer risk: the Swedish follow-up study. *Br J Dermatol* 141(1): 108–112
120 Vallat VP, Gilleaudeau P, Battat L, Wolfe J, Nabeya R, Heftler N, Hodak E, Gottlieb AB, Krueger JG (1994) PUVA bath therapy strongly suppresses immunological and epidermal activation in psoriasis: a possible cellular basis for remittive therapy. *J Exp Med* 180: 283–296
121 Fairhurst DA, Ashcroft DM, Griffiths CE (2005) Optimal management of severe plaque form of psoriasis. *Am J Clin Dermatol* 6: 283–294
122 Halpern SM, Anstey AV, Dawe RS, Diffey BL, Farr PM, Ferguson J, Hawk JL, Ibbotson S, McGregor JM, Murphy GM et al. (2000) Guidelines for topical PUVA: a report of a workshop of the British photodermatology group. *Br J Dermatol* 142: 22–31
123 Oxsoralen-ultra capsules package insert
124 Grundmann-Kollmann M, Behrens S, Peter RU, Kerscher M (1999) Treatment of severe recalci-

trant dermatoses of the palms and soles with PUVA-bath *versus* PUVA-cream therapy. *Photodermatol Photoimmunol Photomed* 15: 87–89
125 Schiener R, Gottlober P, Muller B, Williams S, Pillekamp H, Peter RU, Kerscher M (2005) PUVA-gel *versus* PUVA-bath therapy for severe recalcitrant palmoplantar dermatoses. A randomized, single-blinded prospective study. *Photodermatol Photoimmunol Photomed* 21: 62–67
126 Boyvat A, Erdi H, Birol A, Gurgey E (2000) Interaction of commonly used emollients with photochemotherapy. *Photodermatol Photoimmunol Photomed* 16(4): 156–160
127 Birgin B, Fetil E, Ilknur T, Tahsin Gunes A, Ozkan S (2005) Effects of topical petrolatum and salicylic acid upon skin photoreaction to UVA. *Eur J Dermatol* 15: 156–158
128 Hindson C, Diffey B, Lawlor F, Downey A (1983) Dithranol-UV-A phototherapy (DUVA) for psoriasis: a treatment without dressings. *Br J Dermatol* 108(4): 457–460
129 van de Kerkhof PCM (2001) Therapeutic strategies: rotational therapy and combinations. *Clin Dermatol* 26: 356–361
130 Speight EL, Farr PM (1994) Calcipotriol improves the response of psoriasis to PUVA. *Br J Dermatol* 130(1): 79–82
131 Torras H, Aliaga A, Lopez-Estebaranz JL, Hernandez I, Gardeazabal J, Quintanilla E, Mascaro JM (2004) A combination therapy of calcipotriol cream and PUVA reduces the UVA dose and improves the response of psoriasis vulgaris. *J Dermatol Treat* 15: 98–103
132 Frappaz A, Thivolet J (1993) Calcipotriol in combination with PUVA: a randomized double blind placebo study in severe psoriasis. *Eur J Dermatol* 3: 351–354
133 Kokelj F, Plozzer C, Torsello P (1997) Reduction of UV-A radiation induced by calcipotriol in the treatment of vulgar psoriasis with oral psoralen plus UV-A. *Arch Dermatol* 133: 668–669
134 Grundmann-Kollmann M, Behrens S, Krahn G, Leiter U, Ochsendorf F, Kaufmann R, Peter RU, Kerscher M (1999) Treatment of psoriasis with calcipotriene plus psoralen-UV-A-bath therapy. *Arch Dermatol* 135(7): 861–862
135 Tzaneva S, Honigsmann H, Tanew A, Seeber A (2002) A comparison of psoralen plus ultraviolet A (PUVA) monotherapy, tacalcitol plus PUVA and tazarotene plus PUVA in patients with chronic plaque-type psoriasis. *Br J Dermatol* 147(4): 748–753
136 Glaser R, Rowert J, Mrowietz U (1998) Hyperpigmentation due to topical calcipotriol and photochemotherapy in two psoriatic patients. *Br J Dermatol* 139: 148–151
137 Scott LJ, Dunn CJ, Goa KL (2001) Calcipotriol ointment. A review of its use in the management of psoriasis. *Am J Clin Dermatol* 2: 95–120
138 Youn JI, Park BS, Chung JH, Lee JH (1997) Photoprotective effect of calcipotriol upon skin photoreaction to UVA and UVB. *Photodermatol Photoimmunol Photomed* 13(3): 109–114
139 Lebwohl M, Quijije J, Gilliard J, Rollin T, Watts O (2003) Topical calcitriol is degraded by ultraviolet light. *J Invest Dermatol* 121(3): 594–595
140 Lebwohl M, Hecker D, Martinez J, Sapadin A, Patel B (1997) Interactions between calcipotriene and ultraviolet light. *J Am Acad Dermatol* 37(1): 93–95
141 Behrens S, Grundmann-Kollmann M, Peter RU, Kerscher M (1999) Combination treatment of psoriasis with photochemotherapy and tazarotene gel, a receptor-selective topical retinoid. *Br J Dermatol* 141: 177
142 Schmoll M, Henseler T, Christophers E (1978) Evaluation of PUVA, topical corticosteroids and the combination of both in the treatment of psoriasis. *Br J Dermatol* 99: 693–702
143 Del Rosso J, Friedlander SF (2005) Corticosteroids: Options in the era of steroid-sparing therapy. *J Am Acad Dermatol* 53: S50–S58
144 Tanew A, Guggenbichler A, Honigsmann H, Geiger JM, Fritsch P (1991) Photochemotherapy for severe psoriasis without or in combination with acitretin: a randomized, double-blind comparison study. *J Am Acad Dermatol* 25(4): 682–684
145 Saurat JH, Geiger JM, Amblard P, Beani JC, Boulanger A, Claudy A, Frenk E, Guilhou JJ, Grosshans E, Merot Y et al. (1988) Randomized double-blind multicenter study comparing acitretin-PUVA, etretinate-PUVA and placebo-PUVA in the treatment of severe psoriasis. *Dermatologica* 177(4): 218–224
146 Lauharanta J, Juvakoski T, Lassus A (1981) A clinical evaluation of the effects of an aromatic retinoid (Tigason), combination of retinoid and PUVA, and PUVA alone in severe psoriasis. *Br J Dermatol* 104(3): 325–332
147 Vaatainen N, Hollmen A, Fraki JE (1985) Trimethylpsoralen bath plus ultraviolet A combined with oral retinoid (etretinate) in the treatment of severe psoriasis. *J Am Acad Dermatol* 12: 52–55
148 Muchenberger S, Schof E, Simon JC (1997) The combination of oral acitretin and bath PUVA for

the treatment of severe psoriasis. *Br J Dermatol* 137: 587–589
149 Lebwohl M (2000) Advances in psoriasis therapy. *Dermatol Clin* 18: 13–19
150 Lebwohl M, Tannis C, Carrasco D (2003) Acitretin suppression of squamous cell carcinoma. *J Dermatol Treat* 14(s2): 3–6
151 Morison WL, Momtaz K, Parrish JA, Fitzpatrick TB (1982) Combined methotrexate-PUVA therapy in the treatment of psoriasis. *J Am Acad Dermatol* 6: 46–51
152 Shehzad T, Dar NR, Zakria M (2004) Efficacy of concomitant use of PUVA and methotrexate in disease clearance time in plaque type psoriasis. *J Pakistan Med Assoc* 54(9): 453–455
153 Stern RS, Laird N (1994) The carcinogenic risk of treatments for severe psoriasis. Photochemotherapy Follow-up Study. *Cancer* 73(11): 2759–2764
154 LeVine MJ (1981) Erythema resulting from suberythemogenic doses of ultraviolet radiation and methotrexate. *Arch Dermatol* 117(10): 656–658
155 Hunt MJ, Lee SH, Salisbury EL, Wills EJ, Armati R (1997) Generalized pustular psoriasis responsive to PUVA and oral cyclosporin therapy. *Australas J Dermatol* 38(4): 199–201
156 Petzelbauer P, Honigsmann H, Langer K, Anegg B, Strohal R, Tanew A, Wolff K (1990) Cyclosporin A in combination with photochemotherapy (PUVA) in the treatment of psoriasis. *Br J Dermatol* 123(5): 641–647
157 Marcil I, Stern RS (2001) Squamous-cell cancer of the skin in patients given PUVA and ciclosporin: nested cohort crossover study. *Lancet* 358: 1042–1045
158 Paul CF, Ho VC, McGeown C, Christophers E, Schmidtmann B, Guillaume JC, Lamarque V, Dubertret L (2003) Risk of malignancies in psoriasis patients treated with cyclosporine: a 5 y cohort study. *J Invest Dermatol* 120(2): 211–216
159 Dawe RS (2003) Ultraviolet A phototherapy. *Br J Dermatol* 148: 626–637
160 Godar DE (1999) UVA1 radiation triggers two different final apoptotic pathways. *J Invest Dermatol* 112: 3–12
161 Kowalzick L, Suckow M, Waldmann T, Ponnighaus J-M (1999) Mediumdose UV-A1 *versus* broad-band UV-B in psoriasis. *Z Dermatol* 185: 92–94
162 Tuchinda C, Kerr HA, Taylor CR, Jacobe H, Bergamo BM, Elmets C, Rivard J, Lim HW (2006) UVA1 phototherapy for cutaneous diseases: an experience of 92 cases in the United States. *Photodermatol Photoimmunol Photomed* 22: 247–253
163 Rivard J, Janiga J, Lim HW (2006) Tacrolimus ointment 0.1% alone and in combination with medium-dose UVA1 in the treatment of palmar or plantar psoriasis. *J Drug Dermatol* 5(6): 505–510
164 Roussaki-Schulze AV, Kouskoukis C, Klimi E, Zafiriou E, Galanos A, Rallis E (2005) Calcipotriol monotherapy *versus* calcipotriol plus UVA1 *versus* calcipotriol plus narrow-band UVB in the treatment of psoriasis. *Drugs Exp Clin Res* 31: 169–174
165 Boer J, Schothorst AA, Suurmond D (1981) Influence of UVA on the erythematogenic and therapeutic effects of UVB irradiation in psoriasis; photoaugmentation effects. *J Invest Dermatol* 76(1): 56–58
166 Momtaz-T K, Parrish JA (1984) Combination of psoralens and ultraviolet A and ultraviolet B in the treatment of psoriasis vulgaris: a bilateral comparison study. *J Am Acad Dermatol* 10(3): 481–486
167 Calzavara-Pinton P (1998) Narrow band UVB (311 nm) phototherapy and PUVA photochemotherapy: a combination. *J Am Acad Dermatol* 38(5 Pt 1): 687–690
168 Grundmann-Kollmann M, Ludwig R, Zollner TM, Ochsendorf F, Thaci D, Boehncke WH, Krutmann J, Kaufmann R, Podda M (2004) Narrowband UVB and cream psoralen-UVA combination therapy for plaque-type psoriasis. *J Am Acad Dermatol* 50(5): 734–739
169 Su J, Pearce DJ, Feldman SR (2005) The role of commercial tanning beds and ultraviolet A light in the treatment of psoriasis. *J Dermatol Treatment* 16(5/6): 324–326
170 Griffiths CE, Clark CM, Chalmers RJ, Li Wan Po A, Williams HC (2000) A systematic review of treatments for severe psoriasis. *Health Technology Assessment* (Winchester, England) 4(40): 1–125
171 Koo J, Bandow G, Feldman SR (2003) The art and practice of UVB phototherapy for the treatment of psoriasis. In: GD Weinstein, AB Gottleib (eds): *Therapy of moderate-to-severe psoriasis*. Marcel Dekker Inc, New York, 68–69
172 Ortonne JP, Khemis A, Koo JYM, Choi J (2005) An open-label study of alefacept plus ultraviolet B light as combination therapy for chronic plaque psoriasis. *J Eur Acad Dermatol Venereol* 19: 556–563

173 Scheinfeld N (2005) Therapy-resistant psoriasis treated with alefacept and subsequent narrow band ultraviolet B photo therapy with total clearing of psoriasis. *Dermatol Online J* 11(2): 7
174 Gottlieb AB, Hamilton T, Caro I, Kwon P, Compton PG, Leonardi CL, Efalizumab Study Group (2006) Long-term continuous efalizumab therapy in patients with moderate to severe chronic plaque psoriasis: updated results from an ongoing trial. *J Am Acad Dermatol* 54(4 Suppl 1): S154–163
175 Moore A, Wright E, Ostrowski L, Moore T (2006) Etanercept and narrowband UVB combination therapy for plaque-type psoriasis shortens onset of action in both adults and children. *J Am Acad Dermatol* 54(3 Suppl 1): AB217
176 Yosipovitch G, Tang MBY (2002) Practical management of psoriasis in the elderly: epidemiology, clinical aspects, quality of life, patient education and treatment options. *Drugs Aging* 19(11): 847–863
177 Jury CS, McHenry P, Burden AD, Lever R, Bilsland D (2006) Narrowband ultraviolet B (UVB) phototherapy in children. *Clin Exp Dermatol* 31(2): 196–199
178 Pasic A, Ceovic R, Lipozencic J, Husar K, Susic SM, Skerlev M, Hrsan D (2003) Phototherapy in pediatric patients. *Pediatric Dermatol* 20(1): 71–77
179 Stern RS, Nichols KT (1996) Therapy with orally administered methoxsalen and ultraviolet A radiation during childhood increases the risk of basal cell carcinoma. The PUVA Follow-up Study. *J Pediatrics* 129(6): 915–917
180 Holme SA, Anstey AV (2004) Phototherapy and PUVA photochemotherapy in children. *Photodermatol Photoimmunol Photomed* 20(2): 69–75
181 Pasic A, Ceovic R, Lipozencic J, Husar K, Susic SM, Skerlev M, Hrsan D (2003) Phototherapy in pediatric patients. *Pediatric Dermatol* 20(1): 71–77
182 Tauscher AE, Fleischer AB, Phelps KC, Feldman SR (2002) Psoriasis and pregnancy. *J Cutan Med Surg* 6(6): 561–570
183 Stern RS, Lange R (1991) Outcomes of pregnancies among women and partners of men with a history of exposure to methoxsalen photochemotherapy (PUVA) for the treatment of psoriasis. *Arch Dermatol* 127(3): 347–350
184 Lebwohl M (2005) A clinician's paradigm in the treatment of psoriasis. *J Am Acad Dermatol* 53(1): S59–S69
185 Smit JV, de Jong EM, van Hooijdonk CA, Otero ME, Boezeman JB, van de Kerkhof PC (2004) Systemic treatment of psoriatic patients with bexarotene decreases epidermal proliferation and parameters for inflammation, and improves differentiation in lesional skin. *J Am Acad Dermatol* 51(2): 257–264
186 Smit JV, Franssen ME, de Jong EM, Lambert J, Roseeuw DI, De Weert J, Yocum RC, Stevens VJ, van De Kerkhof PC (2004) A phase II multicenter clinical trial of systemic bexarotene in psoriasis. *J Am Acad Dermatol* 51(2): 249–256
187 Smit JV, De Jong EM, Van De Kerkhof PC (2003) Effects of oral bexarotene (targretin) on the minimal erythema dose for broadspectrum UVB light. *Skin Pharmacol Appl Skin Physiol* 16(4): 237–241
188 Magliocco MA, Pandya K, Dombrovskiy V, Christiansen L, Wong Y, Gottlieb AB (2006) A randomized, double-blind, vehicle-controlled, bilateral comparison trial of bexarotene gel 1% *versus* vehicle gel in combination with narrowband UVB phototherapy for moderate to severe psoriasis vulgaris. *J Am Acad Dermatol* 54(1): 115–118
189 Smits T, Kleinpenning MM, van Erp PEJ, van de Kerkhof PCM, Gerritsen MJP (2006) A placebo controlled randomized study on the clinical effectiveness, immunohistochemical changes and protoporphyrin IX accumulation in fractionated 5-aminolaevulinic acid-photodynamic therapy patients with psoriasis. *Br J Dermatol* 155: 429–436
190 Beattie PE, Dawe RS, Ferguson J, Ibboston SH (2004) Lack of efficacy and tolerability of topical PDT for psoriasis in comparison with narrowband UVB phototherapy. *Clinical Exper Dermatol* 29: 545–562
191 Morton CA, Brown SB, Collins S, Ibbotson S, Jenkinson H, Kurwa H, Langmack K, McKenna K, Moseley H, Pearse AD et al. (2002) Guidelines for topical photodynamic therapy: report of a workshop of the British Photodermatology Group. *Br J Dermatol* 146: 552–567
192 Ibbotson SH (2002) Topical 5-aminolaevulinic acid photodynamic therapy for the treatment of skin conditions other than non-melanoma skin cancer. *Br J Dermatol* 146: 178–188

Treatment of Psoriasis
Edited by J.M. Weinberg

Traditional systemic therapy I: methotrexate and cyclosporine

Edward M. Prodanovic and Neil J. Korman

Department of Dermatology, Murdough Family Center for Psoriasis, University Hospitals Case Medical Center, 11100 Euclid Ave, Cleveland, OH 44106, USA

Many medications have been discovered for the treatment of psoriasis, with methotrexate and cyclosporine being the earliest treatment options. They are complex structures that have shown efficacy, but both carry possible side effects and complications.

Methotrexate

Introduction

Methotrexate (MTX) is an effective agent in the treatment of psoriasis [1], including pustular psoriasis, psoriatic erythroderma, psoriatic arthritis and for extensive chronic plaque psoriasis not controlled by conventional therapy [2–6]. Methotrexate is usually reserved for patients with moderate to severe disease who have at least 5% of their skin covered with psoriasis who are not responsive to, or eligible for, topical or ultraviolet light treatments (including UVB and PUVA) [2–7]. It is critical that physicians prescribing MTX be familiar with its action and potential toxicities.

History

Anti-metabolites mimic substances required for normal biochemical reactions and thus interfere with normal functions of the cell, including cell division. They may masquerade as purines (e.g., azathioprine), pyrimidines (e.g., 5-flourouracil) and folic acid analogs essential for purine and pyrimidine synthesis, (e.g., methotrexate).

MTX, formerly known as aminopterin, has been widely used in the treatment of cancer and autoimmune diseases [8, 9]. It was first developed in the 1940s when scientists were investigating the effects of folic acid on cancer, particularly childhood leukemia [10]. Methotrexate is an analog of folic acid that inhibits cellular proliferation inducing folate coenzyme deficiencies [11].

Mechanism of action

MTX inhibits dihydrofolate reductase (DHFR), which is required to produce tetrahydrofolic acid, the active from of folate in humans. Folate is essential for purine and pyrimidine synthesis and thus for the replication of DNA. Methotrexate acts on this enzyme binding to it some 1'000 times more tightly than folate itself resulting in a substantial negative effect on rapidly dividing cells, including cancer cells [12]. When MTX was incidentally noted to improve psoriatic lesions in the 1960s [2], it became clear that it possessed anti-inflammatory properties in addition to its antiproliferative effects [13–15]. Inhibition of DHFR is more relevant to high dose MTX regimens used in cancer therapy, however low dose MTX therapy appears to inhibit enzymes involved in purine metabolism, leading to an accumulation of adenosine, which has anti-inflammatory properties [16, 17]. A recent study reported that MTX significantly inhibits proliferating lymphoid tissue, particularly T lymphocytes, rather than epidermal cells, i.e., keratinocytes, during low dose once weekly therapy [2, 18]. MTX inhibits T cell activation and suppresses the intercellular adhesion molecule expression by T cells [11]. Interleukin-1 (IL-1), a critical inflammatory cytokine, has some structural similarity to DHFR and it appears to inhibit IL-1 binding to T cell receptors [19, 20].

Pharmacokinetics

The bioavailability of MTX is generally high (approximately 70%), however there is considerable inter-individual variability (between 17–90%). The onset of action of methotrexate usually occurs within 3–6 weeks of the initiation of therapy [21]. MTX is primarily excreted by the kidneys (~90%), whereas 10% is excreted in bile and feces. The elimination half-life of methotrexate is 3–10 h for the low dose therapy that is used to treat psoriasis [22–24].

Initiating and monitoring therapy

Before initiating therapy with methotrexate, patients should have a thorough history and physical exam, reviewing alcohol intake, possible exposure to hepatitis B or C, and family history of liver disease. Laboratory tests, including a complete blood count with differential, serum electrolytes, creatinine, liver function tests including albumin and bilirubin, should be obtained for baseline levels. Screening for hepatitis B and C is recommended if risk factors exist as this would contraindicate the use of MTX. Pretreatment liver biopsy should be performed in patients who have abnormal liver function tests, patients with chronic hepatitis, and patients with a history of significant alcohol intake. A chest radiograph is particularly important for patients with underlying pulmonary disease. Additionally, it is very important to discuss appropriate contraception, as methotrexate therapy during pregnancy is known to increase the risk of serious birth defects [21–25].

Due to the well recognized potential for methotrexate to suppress the bone marrow [26], weekly complete blood count with differential (CBC/diff) is recommended for the first 8 weeks of therapy, followed by every other week for the next 8 weeks of therapy and then every month as long as the patient is taking MTX [25]. Liver function tests should be performed at monthly intervals throughout the course of therapy. If transaminases levels are abnormal or there is an unexplained drop in serum albumin below the normal range, an adjustment of the weekly dose of MTX is advised with repeat blood testing in 2–4 weeks [25, 27]. If liver function tests remain elevated, a liver biopsy is indicated. The extent of fibrosis on liver biopsy dictates whether MTX can be continued. If a patient refuses to undergo a liver biopsy, it is prudent to discontinue MTX [25, 27].

More frequent monitoring of both laboratory studies and liver histology should be performed if other hepatotoxic medications are used along with methotrexate.

Dosage/administration

MTX is usually administered in an intermittent low-dose once weekly regimen. Administration can be oral, intramuscular or subcutaneous. The usual dose range is between 10–25 mg per week until adequate response is achieved [25, 28].

Folic acid, given 1 mg daily 6 of 7 days of the week, protects against some of the common side effects seen with low-dose MTX including stomatitis, hepatotoxicity and gastrointestinal intolerance [29]. It, however, does not appear to protect against pulmonary toxicity. Although folic acid treatment decreases the incidence of hepatotoxicity, it is still appropriate to monitor for both bone marrow suppression and hepatotoxicity during methotrexate therapy in patients being treated with folic acid [25, 29]. Folinic acid should only be used in patients who have not had a satisfactory response to folic acid.

Side effects

60–90% of patients treated with MTX develop minor adverse reactions, including gastrointestinal distress (nausea, vomiting, diarrhea, or anorexia), stomatitis, headaches, and fatigue [15]. These adverse reactions tend to occur within 48 h after the weekly dose.

Severe potentially life threatening toxicities of methotrexate include myelosuppression, hepatotoxicity, and pulmonary damage. These toxicities occur at a significantly higher frequency in patients treated with high dose methotrexate used to treat malignancy, but can also occur with chronic low dose weekly therapy used to treat inflammatory diseases such as psoriasis. Up to 30% of patients treated with chronic low dose MTX for more than 5 years need to discontinue therapy due to the development of serious toxicities [15].

Myelosuppression
With low dose weekly therapy, pancytopenia may be observed. This is more likely in the elderly and with overdose or drug interactions. Furthermore, renal function impairment results in sustained serum levels of MTX that can result in bone marrow toxicity [26, 30].

Hepatotoxicity
Most of the current understanding of the hepatotoxic potential of MTX comes from its use in psoriasis [31, 32]. Hepatotoxicity manifests as fibrosis of increasing severity, which may culminate in cirrhosis. The exact mechanism of hepatotoxicity is still unclear. Several studies have demonstrated that liver function tests may inadequately predict actual liver toxicity, leading to the recommendation for a liver biopsy after a total cumulative dose of 1.5 g of MTX, and again after each additional 1.5 g of cumulative dose [25, 31]. However when rheumatologists began using MTX for rheumatoid arthritis [33], they observed that abnormal transaminase elevations were predictive of worsening abnormal histology on liver biopsy and only minimal differences were noted on serial liver biopsies once MTX was adjusted for abnormal AST and albumin [34, 35]. The difference in hepatotoxicity seen between dermatologists treating patients with psoriasis and rheumatologists treating patients with rheumatoid arthritis are not fully understood. It is however plausible that these differences may be related to differences in the underlying disease processes between psoriasis and rheumatoid arthritis. Another factor that may explain the differences in liver toxicity between psoriasis and rheumatoid arthritis is that psoriasis patients tend to be overweight when compared with rheumatoid arthritis patients and that overweight patients have an increased risk of fatty liver. Recent studies have suggested that monitoring aminoterminal peptide of type III procollagen (PIIINP) levels as a marker for hepatic fibrosis could reduce or possibly eliminate the need for liver biopsies in patients treated with methotrexate and in whom liver biopsy may be contraindicated [36].

Pulmonary toxicity
Methotrexate pneumonitis is rarely seen in patients receiving low dose weekly treatment for psoriasis but it does occur and it can be fatal [37]. In patients given methotrexate for rheumatoid arthritis, the prevalence of pneumonitis is about 5% [37, 38]. Since there is no specific population at risk for this effect and chest x-rays have not proven to be a useful screening tool, it is not necessary to per-

form a chest x-ray unless a patient on therapy develops suggestive symptoms including dyspnea, nonproductive cough, fever or malaise [39]. Immediate withdrawal of methotrexate is imperative if pneumonitis is suspected and some suggest that treatment with systemic corticosteroids is appropriate for patients with methotrexate pneumonitis as long as bacterial infection is ruled out [37].

Infections and malignancies

Since methotrexate works as an immunosuppressive agent by inhibiting lymphocyte function, rare reports of infection and malignancy are not unexpected [40]. However, a clear association between MTX use and malignancy has not been confirmed [41–43].

While there have been many reports of lymphoproliferative disease occurring in rheumatoid arthritis patients treated with methotrexate [44], only rarely has lymphoproliferative disease been associated with methotrexate treatment in patients with psoriasis [45]. Furthermore, a recent study of over 18'000 patients with rheumatoid arthritis did not show an increased standardized incidence ratio of lymphoproliferative disease in patients receiving methotrexate when compared with those who were never exposed to methotrexate [46].

High dose methotrexate therapy is considered a risk factor for the development of non-melanoma skin cancer, particularly squamous cell carcinoma (SCC). However, no studies confirm an increased incidence of SCC in psoriasis patients receiving low-dose methotrexate monotherapy. Conversely, therapy with psoralen and ultraviolet A irradiation (PUVA) significantly increases the overall risk of SCC [47–49].

Contraindications

MTX should not be given to anyone with a history of hypersensitivity to MTX, cytopenia, active liver disease, alcoholism, active infection, or pulmonary hypersensitivity. Renal insufficiency reduces the clearance of MTX and its active metabolites thus increasing the risk of toxicity. Other factors that predispose patients to MTX toxicity include dosing errors, advanced age, untreated folate deficiency, and the use of drugs that block tubular secretion (e.g., probenecid, salicylates) [23, 50].

Pregnancy is an absolute contraindication for treatment with MTX because MTX is teratogenic and multiple congenital deformities have been reported including hydrocephalus, cleft palate, skeletal abnormalities, and abnormal facial features [51, 52]. Adequate contraception (for male as well as female patients) is absolutely necessary while taking MTX. In males, methotrexate can cause reversible oligospermia and defective sperm [53]. Women should not become pregnant for 1 month and men should avoid fathering children for 3 months following cessation of methotrexate therapy [54, 55]. Women should not breastfeed while taking MTX. Patients taking MTX should not receive live virus vaccines.

Use of methotrexate in children

Methotrexate use in childhood psoriasis is scarce and only a few studies with small sample sizes exist that demonstrate some efficacy in children. However there are concerns over long-term safety, particularly its hepatotoxic potential and risk of myleosuppression [56, 57]. Tolerable doses of 0.2–0.4 mg/kg have been used with no detectable hematologic or biochemical abnormalities. However, most of the data regarding the use of methotrexate in pediatric psoriasis has been extrapolated from adult data [58].

Cyclosporine

Introduction

Cyclosporine, which is believed by most dermatologists to be the most effective available oral therapy to treat patients with psoriasis, was originally developed to prevent rejection of organ transplants. Although cyclosporine is generally well tolerated, the safety profile, including the risk of hypertension and nephrotoxicity, supports the use of cyclosporine in patients who either have failed previous treatment or are not candidates for other systemic therapies. Even though cyclosporine is extremely effective in all of the subtypes of psoriasis, including pustular and erythrodermic psoriasis [59, 60], concern about potential side effects and lack of both training and experience have prevented many dermatologists from utilizing this extremely effective therapy.

History

Cyclosporine is a potent immunosuppressive agent that has been widely used in organ transplantation. In 1979, cyclosporine was fortuitously found to clear psoriasis in patients being treated for severe longstanding rheumatoid arthritis [61]. Since the late 1980s, cyclosporine has been successfully used to treat many autoimmune disorders, including rheumatoid arthritis, polymyositis, dermatomyositis, systemic lupus erythematosus, ulcerative colitis, and myasthenia gravis [62–72].

Numerous studies have demonstrated the efficacy of cyclosporine in the treatment of psoriasis [73–75] and in 1997 cyclosporine was FDA approved for the treatment of psoriasis.

Mechanism of action

Cyclosporine is a cyclic peptide of 11 amino acids produced by a fungus, *Tolypocladium inflatum gams* [76]. Cyclosporine has immunosuppressive effects on both cellular and humoral mediated immune responses. Cyclosporine shows preferential binding to a group of cytoplasmic proteins called cyclophilins, in particular cyclophilin A [77].

This complex binds and inhibits calcineurin, an enzyme that normally increases the production of numerous cytokines including interleukin-2 (IL-2), tumor necrosis factor alpha (TNF-alpha), IL-3, IL-4, CD40L, granulocyte-macrophage colony-stimulating factor, and interferon-gamma [78–82].

Cyclophilins have additionally been shown to possess chemotactic activity, recruiting leukocytes such as neutrophils and eosinophils [83]. Although cyclophilins are primarily found in the cytosol of most cells, minimal concentrations have also been discovered in human plasma. Interestingly, elevated plasma levels of cyclophilin A are detected in septic patients, suggesting that it is released during inflammation and/or infection. Furthermore, cyclophilin A accumulation is found in the synovial fluids of patients with rheumatoid arthritis suggesting that it may play a role in the progression of this inflammatory disease [84].

These findings suggest that cyclosporine could act as a direct anti-inflammatory agent by binding to cyclophilins and inhibiting their chemotaxis.

Pharmacokinetics

Oral cyclosporine is lipophilic and undergoes extensive body distribution [85]. The oral bioavailability is limited with intra-individual variability secondary to first-pass hepatic metabolism and partial metabolism by enzymes in the bowel mucosa [86]. Cyclosporine absorption is increased when ingested with fatty meals.

Cyclosporine is metabolized by the cytochrome P450 system in the liver and excreted into the bile. Therefore a variety of important drug interactions can occur with drugs that are also metabolized by these enzymes [85, 87]. Medications such as diltiazem and ketoconazole increase cyclosporine levels which has led to their use in post-transplant patients for lowering the total cyclosporine dose.

The elimination half-life for cyclosporine is 19 h and liver dysfunction prolongs its half-life. Metabolites of cyclosporine have been found to hold between 10–20% of the drug's immunosuppressive activity [85–88].

Initiating and monitoring therapy

A thorough history and physical examination with blood pressure documentation, complete blood count, plasma creatinine level with chemistry panel, and uric acid level should be obtained before starting cyclosporine therapy [87, 89]. Due to the critical importance of accurate measurement of baseline renal function, many authors suggest obtaining daily fasting creatinine level, performed on three consecutive day and then taking the average as the baseline creatinine level.

Blood pressure and a complete metabolic panel that includes electrolytes, magnesium, creatinine, blood urea nitrogen, glucose, and transaminases should be monitored every 2 weeks for the first 3 months of therapy, and every 1 to 2 months thereafter. Hypertension during therapy with cyclosporine should prompt reduction in dosage or initiation of anti-hypertensive therapy. Measurement of the serum creatinine level is used to follow renal function. An increase of the serum creatinine level of more than 30% above baseline requires either a decrease of the dose or a temporary discontinuation of the cyclosporine [87, 90]. However, many experienced clinicians will lower the dosage of cyclosporine if the creatinine rises by 15–20%.

Any changes in the clinical regimen should be made slowly with the lowest effective dose of medication used. It is important to note that clinically important toxicity, e.g., nephrotoxicity, can occur when doses of cyclosporine are within the 'therapeutic range', [90] further underscoring the need for accurate baseline measurement of creatinine.

Dosage/administration

The oral dose of cyclosporine should be based on ideal body weight. Cyclosporine microemulsion (Neoral®, Gengraf®) is preferred to the regular preparation for its superior pharmacokinetic profile and equal price. Cyclosporine should be administered at a consistent time of the day and in relation to meals to decrease the intra-individual blood level variations. The cyclosporine solution can be mixed with milk or orange juice but should not be mixed with grapefruit juice since this can increase plasma cyclosporine concentrations by inhibiting cytochrome P450 metabolism of cyclosporine. Initial daily dose of cyclosporine microemulsion (Neoral®, Gengraf®) is 2.5 mg/kg in two divided doses. The dose can be increased to maximum of 5 mg/kg per day [85, 87].

Although the majority of cyclosporine studies utilize continuous ongoing therapy, this is impractical as the requirement is to discontinue cyclosporine therapy after one year of treatment. Intermittent short (2–3 month) courses of cyclosporine are effective and well tolerated with an improved safety profile compared with continuous cyclosporine monotherapy [91].

Side effects

Nephrotoxicity is the most common and clinically significant adverse effect of cyclosporine [92]. The renal effects of cyclosporine can manifest as acute azotemia (that appears to be dose related and reversible upon discontinuation of the drug), elevated blood pressures, tubular dysfunction, or as chronic progressive renal disease that is irreversible [87, 93, 94].

Cyclosporine causes vasoconstriction of afferent and efferent glomerular arterioles, decreased glomerular filtration rate and reduced renal blood flow [95]. Long-term cyclosporine exposure has been associated with reduction in glomerular filtration rate [96]. Renal biopsies performed on these patients reveal ischemic scarring of the glomeruli, obliterative arteriolopathy suggesting endothelial damage, tubular atrophy and interstitial fibrosis. Fortunately these findings are seen more commonly with high dose cyclosporine therapy [97, 98].

The renal interstitial fibrosis may be mediated by the increased expression of transforming growth factor-beta (TGF-beta), a stimulator of extracellular matrix production [99, 100]. Decreased levels of nitric oxide as well as elevated levels of angiotensin II have been observed to induce TGF-beta production. Improvement of renal insufficiency and hypertension has been observed with angiotensin converting enzyme (ACE) inhibitors and angiotensin II receptor antagonists by minimizing interstitial fibrosis without affecting glomerular or tubular injury [92, 99–102].

One year studies have suggested that the risk of chronic nephrotoxicity is minimized using low dose cyclosporine therapy (less than 5 mg/kg/day) for the treatment of patients with autoimmune diseases. Avoiding increases in serum creatinine of more than 30% above the patient's base-line value will minimize the risk of irreversible and progressive renal dysfunction [103].

Hypertension caused by renal vasoconstriction and sodium retention, is generally seen within the first few weeks of therapy. The prevalence rates of hypertension in patients receiving cyclosporine for psoriasis range from 23–54% [104, 105]. The blood pressure elevation induced by cyclosporine frequently responds to dose reduction, but antihypertensive medications may be required in some patients. Calcium channel blockers are considered the drugs of choice if antihypertensive therapy is needed in the setting of cyclosporine therapy due to their ability to reverse the renal vasoconstriction caused by cyclosporine [105, 106].

Electrolyte disturbances can be seen with cyclosporine use. Reduced efficiency of urinary potassium excretion by directly impairing the function of potassium secreting cells in the collecting tubule can lead to hyperkalemia that can be further exacerbated with use of medications that diminish aldosterone release, such as the ACE inhibitors [107, 108]. Hypomagnesemia can also be seen due to decreased magnesium reabsorption and renal wasting [109].

Cyclosporine's effect on glomeruli and tubules can result in exacerbations of gout due to hyperuricemia as well as a hyperchloremic metabolic acidosis secondary to impaired acid excretion [81, 85].

Neurologic side effects have been reported in patients being treated with cyclosporine with symptoms such as headaches and visual abnormalities, resembling hypertensive encephalopathy [110]. Psychosis, seizures, anxiety and sleep disturbances have been documented but are rare. Most neurologic side effects are reversible with lowering the dose or discontinuing the drug [110–112].

Cyclosporine has been associated with an increased risk of non-melanoma skin cancers, particularly squamous cell carcinoma (SCC). The risk of SCC is higher in patients with greater duration of exposure to cyclosporine. Furthermore, long-term exposure to PUVA significantly adds to the overall risk as does the use of other immunosuppressive therapies [113, 114]. SCC can present as long as 1–2 years after cyclosporine has been discontinued [114]. It is recommended to screen patients with psoriasis for cutaneous malignancy before initiating cyclosporine therapy. Lymphoproliferative disorders have rarely been reported with use of cyclosporine [115, 116]. Spontaneous regression of the lymphoproliferative disorder has occurred when cyclosporine is discontinued since the cumulative level of immunosuppression appears to increase the risk of malignancy. The greater carcinogenic effect of cyclosporine in contrast to methotrexate may be due to direct cellular effects that promote cancer progression in addition to its immunosuppressive action [113]. The results of animal studies suggest that cyclosporine's stimulation of TGF-beta may promote cancer progression [117].

Other potential side effects of cyclosporine include gastrointestinal symptoms such as anorexia, nausea, vomiting, diarrhea and abdominal discomfort [85, 87], and gingival hyperplasia with higher doses of cyclosporine therapy and poor dental hygiene. Case reports have suggested that gingival hyperplasia can be effectively treated with a short course of metronidazole or azithromycin [118–120].

Unlike other immunosuppressive agents, cyclosporine lacks clinically significant myelosuppression [121].

Prevention of chronic cyclosporine nephrotoxicity

There is much interest in developing therapeutic strategies that minimize the nephrotoxic effects of cyclosporine. No agent has thus far been clearly effective. Omega-3 fatty acids were introduced since they may reduce expression of cytokines and thromboxane synthesis diminishing cyclosporine induced vasoconstriction and hypertension. However, only a modest benefit was reported in the studies performed on renal transplant patients [122–124].

Calcium channel blockers do appear to minimize renal vasoconstriction, however may not prevent chronic vascular and tubulointerstitial injury [125–127]. When ACE inhibitors are compared to calcium channel blockers, there are no significant differences in renal function even though ACE inhibitors are considered renal protective by a different mechanism [102, 128].

Thromboxane synthesis inhibitors have been evaluated for their potential role in blocking cyclosporine induced renal vasoconstriction without any clinically significant findings [129].

Contraindications

Hypersensitivity to cyclosporine, current systemic malignancy (except for non-melanoma skin cancer), uncontrolled hypertension, renal insufficiency, and uncontrolled infections are all contraindications for use of cyclosporine. Cyclosporine can be used cautiously in the elderly, immunodeficient, obese, and/or pregnant patients. Furthermore, care should be taken when using other medications that may interact with cyclosporine [85, 87].

Use of cyclosporine in children

Systemic treatment is usually reserved for the management of children with severe subtypes of psoriasis who have not responded to topical and phototherapy. Many clinicians use retinoids but regular monitoring of lipid profiles, liver enzymes and growth parameters are important. Skeletal complications such as premature closure of epiphysis and calcification of ligaments and tendons have been reported and may be irreversible if not caught early [130]. Adverse mucocutaneous reactions are not common with retinoids and include lip xerosis, epistaxis and generalized dry skin [131].

Though cyclosporine has not been extensively studied in pediatric psoriasis, there are studies which demonstrate its efficacy and relative safety in pediatric atopic dermatitis [132, 133] and in organ transplant patients [134]. Most serious side effects, hypertension and nephrotoxicity, can be controlled by dose adjustments and pharmacological intervention. The dosage for childhood psoriasis has been extrapolated from adult data. Initial doses between 2–4 mg/kg/day with titration up to 5 mg/kg/day after 6–8 weeks of therapy have shown good response. Some data has shown pharmacokinetic differences between pediatric and adult populations suggesting lower oral absorption, rapid clearance and greater volume of distribution at a steady state in children [135, 136]. Although these theoretical concerns suggest that the treatment of pediatric psoriasis with cyclosporine may require higher dosing, most clinical studies demonstrate that doses of 2.5–5 mg/kg/day are effective [132]. Cyclosporine may be considered as an alternative treatment when other therapies are unsuccessful.

Use of cyclosporine in pregnancy

There are conflicting reports on the transfer of cyclosporine across the placenta [137]. Cyclosporine appears to lack teratogenic effects, however prematurity and growth restriction were observed in about 40% of neonates born to mothers with organ transplants who were on cyclosporine. The use of cyclosporine in pregnancy should only be considered when the potential benefits outweigh the risk to the fetus. The long-term effects of children who have been exposed to cyclosporine *in utero* is an area of active investigation [138, 139]. The use of cyclosporine during breastfeeding is not recommended [140].

Comparison of the efficacy of methotrexate and cyclosporine

Successful treatment of patients with psoriasis who are candidates for systemic therapy has been clearly demonstrated with both methotrexate and cyclosporine use. Methotrexate data, mainly derived from retrospective studies and case reports, shows reduction of the severity of psoriasis by at least 50–60% in about three quarters of patients within 4–6 months [141, 142]. Cyclosporine efficacy has been documented in many studies; however there is variability of results reported due to different cyclosporine doses, duration of treatments, sample sizes, and outcomes used. Despite these discrepancies, between 50–80% of patients achieve a 75% improvement after 8 weeks and 16 weeks of treatment, respectively [142, 143].

While it is difficult to find a well-designed, randomized trial that evaluates the efficacy of methotrexate *versus* cyclosporine, one study compared these two therapies [144]. A total of 88 patients with moderate to severe psoriasis were randomly assigned for 16 weeks to either methotrexate or cyclosporine. The initial doses utilized were 15 mg per week and 3 mg/kg per day of methotrexate and cyclosporine, respectively, with dose escalation as required. The primary outcome in this study was the difference in the Psoriasis Area and Severity Index (PASI), a well accepted clinical measure of psoriasis severity. The results demonstrated that 64% of methotrexate treated patients and 72% of the cyclosporine treated patients achieved a PASI-75 response at 16 weeks. 12 patients in the methotrexate group had to discontinue therapy because of elevations in liver function tests, and one patient in the cyclosporine group had to discontinue therapy due to an elevated bilirubin level. Overall, both methotrexate and cyclosporine led to improvement of psoriasis with similar efficacies [144]. This is the one of the first studies to compare two effective therapies for psoriasis in a randomized, controlled, clinical trial. Roughly 64% and 40% of patients treated with methotrexate and 72% and 33% of patients treated with cyclosporine achieved partial and nearly complete remission, respectively. Relapse occurred within 4 weeks of cessation of both methotrexate and cyclosporine. Although longer term studies will be necessary to compare and quantify the frequency and character of the toxic effects of methotrexate and cyclosporine, this study yields valuable short-term comparison information on the use of both cyclosporine and methotrexate in the treatment of psoriasis.

References

1 Ryan TJ, Vickers HR, Salem SN, Callender ST, Badenoch J (1964) The treatment of psoriasis with folic acid antagonist. *Br J Dermatol* 76: 555–564

2 Boffa M, Chalmers R (1996) Methotrexate for psoriasis. *Clin Exp Dermatol* 21: 399–408
3 Ryan TJ, Baker H (1969) Systemic corticosteroids and folic acid antagonists in the treatment of generalized pustular psoriasis: evaluation and prognosis based on the study of 104 cases. *Br J Dermatol* 81: 134–145
4 Rosenbaum MM, Roenigk HH Jr, (1984) Treatment of generalized pustular psoriasis with etretinate and methotrexate. *J Am Acad Dermatol* 102: 357–361
5 Black RL, O'Brien WM, Van Scott EJ, Auerbach R, Eisen AZ, Bunim JJ (1964) Methotrexate therapy in psoriatic arthritis. *J Am Med Assoc* 189: 743–747
6 Espinoza LR, Zakraoui L, Espinoza CG, Gutierrez F, Jara LJ, Silveira LH, Cuellar ML, Martinez-Osuna P (1992) Psoriatic arthritis: clinical response and side effects to methotrexate therapy. *J Rheumatol* 19: 872–877
7 Bright R (1999) Methotrexate in the treatment of psoriasis. *Cutis* 64: 332–334
8 Seeger DR, Cosalich DDB, Smith JM, Hultquist ME (1949) Analogs of pteroylglutamic acid. II. 4-aminoderivatives. *J Am Chem Soc* 71: 1297–1301
9 Gubner R, August S, Ginsberg V (1951) Therapeutic suppression of tissue reactivity. II. Effect of aminopterin in rheumatoid arthritis and psoriasis. *Am J Med Sci* 221: 176–182
10 Ward JR (1985) Historical perspective on the use of methotrexate for the treatment of rheumatoid arthritis. *J Rheum* 12: 3–6
11 Cronstein BN (1996) Molecular therapeutics: Methotrexate and its mechanism of action. *Arthritis Rheum* 39: 1951–1960
12 Goodsell DS (1999) The molecular perspective: Methotrexate. *The Oncologist* 4: 430–441
13 Lynch JP 3rd, McCune J (1997) Immunosuppressive and cytotoxic pharmacotherapy for pulmonary disorders. *Am J Respir Crit Care Med* 155: 395–420
14 Kremer JM (1996) Methotrexate update. *Scand J Rheumatol* 25: 341–344
15 Goodman TA, Polisson RP (1994) Methotrexate: Adverse reactions and major toxicities. *Rheum Dis Clin North Am* 20: 513–528
16 Cronstein BN, Naime D, Ostad E (1993) The anti-inflammatory mechanism of methotrexate: increased adenosine release at inflamed sites diminishes leukocyte accumulation in an *in vivo* model of inflammation. *J Clin Invest* 92: 2675–2682
17 Bouma MG, Stad RK, van der Wildenberg FA, Buuman WA (1994) Differential regulatory effects of adenosine on cytokine release by activated human monocytes. *J Immunol* 153: 4159–4168
18 Jeffes EWB, McCullough JL, Pittelkow MR, McCormick A, Almanzor J, Liu G, Dang M, Voss K, Voss J, Schlotzhauer A (1995) Methotrexate therapy of psoriasis: differential sensitivity of proliferating lymphoid and epithelial cells to the cytotoxic and growth-inhibitory effects of methotrexate. *J Invest Dermatol* 104: 183–188
19 Miller LC, Cohen FE, Orencole SF, Schaller JG, Savage N, Dinarello CA (1988) Interleukin-1 beta is structurally related to dihydrofolate reductase: effects of methotrexate on IL-1. *Lymphokine Res* 7: 272A
20 Brody M, Bohm I, Bauer R (1993) Mechanism of action of methotrexate: experimental evidence that methotrexate blocks the binding of interleukin 1 beta to the interleukin 1 receptor on target cells. *Eur J Chem Clin Biochem* 31: 667–674
21 Olsen EA (1991) The pharmacology of methotrexate. *J Am Acad Dermatol* 25: 306–618
22 Jolivet J, Cowan KH, Curt GA, Clendeninn NJ, Chabner BA (1983) The pharmacology and clinical use of methotrexate. *N Engl J Med* 309: 1094–1104
23 Thomson Micromedex Healthcare Series. The Drugpoint summary for methotrexate. Available at: http://www.micromedex.com (accessed 23 January 2007)
24 Huffman DH, Wan SH, Azarnoff DL, Hoogstraten B (1973) Pharmacokinetics of methotrexate. *Clin Pharmacol Ther* 14: 572–579
25 Roenigk HH Jr, Auerbach R, Maibach H, Weinstein G, Lebwohl M (1998) Methotrexate in psoriasis: Consensus conference. *J Am Acad Dermatol* 38: 478–485
26 Singh Y, Aggarwal A, Misra R, Agarwal V (2007) Low-dose methotrexate-induced pancytopenia. *Clin Rheumatol* 26: 84–87
27 Kremer HM, Phelps CT, Lightfoot RW Jr, Willkens RF, Furst DE, Williams HJ, Dent PB, Weinblatt ME (1994) Methotrexate for rheumatoid arthritis. Suggested guidelines for monitoring liver toxicity. American College of Rheumatology. *Arthritis Rheum* 37: 316–328
28 Weinstein GD, Frost P (1971) Methotrexate for psoriasis – a new therapeutic schedule. *Arch Dermatol* 103: 33–38

29 Strober BE, Menon K (2005) Folate supplementation during methotrexate therapy for patients with psoriasis. *J Am Acad Dermatol* 53: 652–659
30 Gutierrez-Urena S, Molina JF, Garcia CO, Cuellar ML, Espinoza LR (1996) Pancytopenia secondary to methotrexate therapy in rheumatoid arthritis. *Arthritis Rheum* 39: 272
31 Weinstein GD, Roenigk H, Maibach HI, Cosmides J, Halprin K, Millard M (1973) Psoriasis-liver-methotrexate interactions. *Arch Dermatol* 108: 36–42
32 Nyfors A (1977) Liver biopsies from psoriatics related to methotrexate therapy: 3. Findings in post-methotrexate liver biopsies from 160 psoriatics. *Acta Pathol Microbiol Scand* 85: 511–518
33 Furst DE, Kremer JM (1988) Methotrexate in rheumatoid arthritis. *Arthritis Rheum* 31: 305–314
34 Kremer JM, Kaye GI, Kaye NW, Ishak KG, Axiotis CA (1995) Light and electron microscope analysis of sequential liver biopsy samples from rheumatoid arthritis patients receiving longterm methotrexate therapy. Follow up over long treatment intervals and correlation with clinical and laboratory variables. *Arthritis Rheum* 38: 1194–1203
35 Kremer JM, Furst ED, Weinblatt ME, Blotner SD (1996) Significant changes in serum AST across hepatic histological biopsy grades: prospective analysis of 3 cohorts receiving methotrexate therapy for rheumatoid arthritis. *J Rheumatol* 23: 459–461
36 Maurice PD, Maddox AJ, Green CA, Tatnall F, Schofield JK, Stott DJ (2005) Monitoring patients on methotrexate: hepatic fibrosis not seen in patients with normal serum assays of aminoterminal peptide of type III procollagen. *Br J Dermatol* 152: 451–458
37 Phillips TJ, Jones DH, Baker H (1987) Pulmonary complications following methotrexate therapy. *J Am Acad Dermatol* 16: 373–375
38 Zitnik RJ, Cooper JA Jr, (1990) Pulmonary disease due to antirheumatic agents. *Clin Chest Med* 11: 139–150
39 Wolverton SE (1991) Systemic drug therapy for psoriasis: the most critical issues. *Arch Dermatol* 127: 565–568
40 Shiroky JB, Frost A, Skelton JD, Hoegert DG, Newkirk MM, Neville C (1991) Complications of immunosuppression associated with weekly low dose methotrexate. *J Rheumatol* 18: 1172–1175
41 Weinblatt ME (1996) Methotrexate in rheumatoid arthritis: toxicity issues. *Br J Rheumatol* 35: 403–405
42 Kamel OW, van de Rijn M, Weiss LM, Del Zoppo GJ, Hench PK, Robbins BA, Montgomery PG, Warnke RA, Dorfman RF (1993) Brief report: Reversible lymphomas associated with Epstein-Barr virus occurring during methotrexate therapy for rheumatoid arthritis and dermatomyositis. *N Engl J Med* 328: 1317–1321
43 Bologna C, Picot MC, Jorgensen C, Viu P, Verdier R, Sany J (1997) Study of 8 cases of cancer in 426 rheumatoid arthritis patients treated with methotrexate. *Ann Rheum Dis* 56: 97–102
44 McClure SL, Valentine J, Gordon KB (2002) Comparative tolerability of systemic treatments for plaque-type psoriasis. *Drug Saf* 25: 913–927
45 Paul C, Le Tourneau A, Cayuela JM, Devidas A, Robert C, Molinie V, Dubertret L (1997) Epstein-Barr virus-associated lymphoproliferative disease during methotrexate therapy for psoriasis. *Arch Dermatol* 133: 867–871
46 Wolfe F, Micahaud K (2004) Lymphoma in rheumatoid arthritis: the effect of methotrexate and anti-tumor necrosis factor therapy in 18'572 patients. *Arthritis Rheum* 50: 1740–1751
47 Stern RS, Laird N (1994) The carcinogenic risk of treatments for severe psoriasis. Photochemotherapy Follow-Up Study. *Cancer* 73: 2759–2764
48 Lindskov R (1983) Skin carcinomas and treatment with photochemotherapy (PUVA). Acta *Derm Venereol* 63: 223–226
49 Stern RS, Zierler S, Parrish JA (1982) Methotrexate used for psoriasis and the risk of noncutaneous or cutaneous malignancy. *Cancer* 50: 869–872
50 Conaghan PG, Quinn DI, Brooks PM, Day RO (1995) Hazards of low dose methotrexate. *Aust N Z J Med* 25: 670–673
51 Buckley LM, Bullaboy CA, Leichtman L, Marquez M (1997) Multiple congenital anomalies associated with weekly low dose methotrexate treatment of the mother. *Arthritis Rheum* 40: 971–973
52 Milunsky A, Graef JW, Gaynor MF Jr, (1968) Methotrexate induces congenital malformations. *J Pediatr* 72: 790–795
53 Georgouras KE, Zagarella SS, Cains GD, Brown PJ (1997) Systemic treatment of severe psoriasis. *Australas J Dermatol* 38: 171–180
54 Jeffes EW 3rd, Weinstein GD (1995) Methotrexate and other chemotherapeutic agents used to treat psoriasis. *Dermatol Clin* 13: 875–890

55 Wolverton SE (1991) Systemic drug therapy for psoriasis: the most critical issues. *Arch Dermatol* 127: 565–568
56 Dogra S, Handa S, Kanwar AJ (2004) Methotrexate in severe childhood psoriasis. *Pediatr Dermatol* 21: 283–284
57 Kumar B, Dhar S, Handa S, Kaur I (1994) Methotrexate in childhood psoriasis. *Pediatr Dermatol* 11: 271–273
58 Leman J, Burden D (2001) Psoriasis in children: a guide to its diagnosis and management. *Paediatr Drugs* 3: 673–680
59 Kapoor R, Kapoor JR (2006) Cyclosporine resolves generalized pustular psoriasis of pregnancy. *Arch Dermatol* 142: 1373–1375
60 Picascia DD, Garden JM, Freinkel RK, Roenigk HH (1987) Treatment of resistant severe psoriasis with systemic cyclosporine. *J Am Acd Dermatol* 17 (3): 480–514
61 Mueller W, Herrmann B (1979) Cyclosporin A for psoriasis. *N Engl J Med* 301: 555
62 Tugwell P, Bombardier C, Gent M, Bennett KJ, Bensen WG, Carette S, Chalmers A, Esdaile JM, Klinkhoff AV, Kraag GR (1990) Low-dose cyclosporine *versus* placebo in patients with rheumatoid arthritis. *Lancet* 335: 1051–1055
63 Bombardier C, Buchbinder R, Tugwell P (1992) Efficacy of cyclosporin A in rheumatoid arthritis: long-term follow-up data and the effect on quality of life. *Scand J Rheumatol* 21: 29–33
64 Pistoia V, Buoncompagni A, Scribanis R, Fasce L, Alpigiani G, Cordone G, Ferrarini M, Borrone C, Cottafava F (1993) Cyclosporin A in the treatment of juvenile chronic arthritis and childhood polymyositis-dermatomyositis. Results of a preliminary study. *Clin Exp Rheumatol* 11: 203–208
65 Reiff A, Rawlings DJ, Shaham B, Franke E, Richardson L, Szer IS, Bernstein BH (1997) Preliminary evidence for cyclosporin A as an alternative in the treatment of recalcitrant juvenile rheumatoid arthritis and juvenile dermatomyositis. *J Rheumatol* 24: 2436–2443
66 Zeller V, Cohen P, Prieur AM, Guillevin L (1996) Cyclosporin A therapy in refractory juvenile dermatomyositis. Experience and long term follow up of 6 cases. *J Rheumatol* 23: 1424–1427
67 Tellus MM, Buchanan RR (1995) Effective treatment of anti Jo-1 antibody-positive polymyositis with cyclosporine. *Br J Rheumatol* 34: 1187–1188
68 Qushmaq KA, Chalmers A, Esdaile JM (2000) Cyclosporin A in the treatment of refractory adult polymyositis/dermatomyositis: population based experience in 6 patients and literature review. *J Rheumatol* 27: 2855–2859
69 Tokuda M, Kurata N, Mizoguchi A, Inoh M, Seto K, Kinashi M, Takahara J (1994) Effect of low-dose cyclosporin A on systemic lupus erythematosus disease activity. *Arthritis Rheum* 37: 551–558
70 Hallegua D, Wallace DJ, Metzger AL, Rinaldi RZ, Klinenberg JR (2000) Cyclosporine for lupus membranous nephritis: experience with ten patients and review of the literature. *Lupus* 9: 241–251
71 Carbonnel F, Boruchovicz A, Duclos B, Soule JC, Lerebours E, Lemann M, Belaiche J, Colombel JF, Cosnes J, Gendre JP (1996) Intravenous cyclosporine in attacks of ulcerative colitis. Short-term and long-term responses. *Dig Dis Sci* 41: 2471–2476
72 Ciafaloni E, Nikhar NK, Massey JM, Sanders DB (2000) Retrospective analysis of the use of cyclosporine in myasthenia gravis. *Neurology* 55: 448–450
73 Fry L (1992) Psoriasis: immunopathology and long-term treatment with cyclosporine. *J Autoimmun* 5: 277–283
74 Mahrle G, Schulze HJ, Farber L, Weidinger G, Steigleder GK (1995) Low-dose short-term cyclosporine *versus* etretinate in psoriasis: improvement of skin, nail, and joint involvement. *J Am Acad Dermatol* 32: 78–88
75 Ellis CN, Fradin MS, Hamiton TA, Voorhees JJ (1995) Duration of remission during maintenance cyclosporine therapy for psoriasis. *Arch Dermatol* 131: 791–795
76 Sneader W (1985) *Drug Discovery: The Evolution of Modern Medicines*. John Wiley, Chichester
77 Handschumacher RE, Harding MW, Rice J, Drugge RJ, Speicher DW (1984) Cyclophilin: a specific cytosolic binding protein for cyclosporin A. *Science* 226: 544–547
78 Wiederrecht G, Lam E, Hung S, Martin M, Sigal N (1993) The mechanism of action of FK506 and cyclosporin A. *Ann NY Acad Sci* 696: 9–19
79 Schreiber SL, Crabtree GR (1992) The mechanism of action of cyclosporin A and FK506. *Immunol Today* 13: 136–142
80 Timmerman LA, Clipstone NA, Ho SN, Northrop JP, Crabtree GR (1996) Rapid shuttling of NF-AT in discrimination of Ca^{2+} signals and immunosuppression. *Nature* 383: 837–840
81 Kahan BD (1989) Drug therapy: Cyclosporine. *N Engl J Med* 321: 1725–1738

82 Klintmalm GB (1994) FK506: an update. *Clin Transplant* 8: 207–210
83 Xu Q, Leiva MC, Fischkoff SA, Handschumacher RE, Lyttle CR (1992) Leukocyte chemotactic activity of cyclophilin. *J Biol Chem* 267: 11968–11971
84 Billich A, Winkler G, Aschauer H, Rot A, Peichl P (1997) Presence of cyclophilin A in synovial fluids of patients with rheumatoid arthritis. *J Exp Med* 185: 975–980
85 Thomson Micromedex Healthcare Series. The Drugpoint summary for cyclosporine. Available at: http://www.micromedex.com (accessed 23 January 2007)
86 Kolars JC, Awni WM, Merion RM, Watkins PB (1991) First-pass metabolism of cyclosporine by the gut. *Lancet* 338: 1488–1490
87 Lebwohl M, Ellis C, Gottlieb A, Koo J, Krueger G, Linden K, Shupack J, Weinstein G (1998) Cyclosporine consensus conference: with emphasis on the treatment of psoriasis. *J Am Acad Dermatol* 39: 464–475
88 Gruber SA, Hewitt JM, Sorenson AL, Barber DL, Bowers L, Rynders G, Arrazola L, Matas AJ, Rosenberg ME, Canafax DM (1994) Pharmacokinetics of FK506 after intravenous and oral administration in patients awaiting renal transplantation. *J Clin Pharmacol* 34: 859–864
89 Panayi GS, Tugwell P (1997) The use of cyclosporin A microemulsion in rheumatoid arthritis: Conclusions of an international review. *Br J Rheumatol* 36: 808–811
90 Berth-Jones J (2005) The use of cyclosporin in psoriasis. *J Dermatolog Treat* 16: 258–277
91 Ho VC, Griffiths CE, Berth-Jones J, Papp KA, Vanaclocha F, Dauden E, Beard A, Puvanarajan L, Paul C (2001) Intermittent short courses of cyclosporine microemulsion for the long-term management of psoriasis: a 2-year cohort study. *J Am Acad Dermatol* 44: 643–651
92 Burdmann EA, Andoh TF, Yu L, Bennett WM (2003) Cyclosporine nephrotoxicity. *Semin Nephrol* 23: 465–476
93 Lamas S (2005) Cellular mechanisms of vascular injury mediated by calcineurin inhibitors. *Kidney Int* 68: 898–907
94 Williams D, Haragsim L (2006) Calcineurin nephrotoxicity. *Adv Chronic Kidney Dis* 13: 47–55
95 Lanese DM, Conger JD (1993) Effects of endothelin receptor antagonist on cyclosporine-induced vasoconstriction in isolated rat renal arterioles. *J Clin Invest* 91: 2144–2149
96 Myers BD, Newton L (1991) Cyclosporine-induced chronic nephropathy: an obliterative microvascular renal injury. *J Am Soc Nephrol* 2: S45–52
97 Di Paolo S, Teutonico A, Stallone G, Infante B, Schena A, Grandaliano G, Battaglia M, Ditonno P, Schena PF (2004) Cyclosporin exposure correlates with 1 year graft function and histological damage in renal transplanted patients. *Nephrol Dial Transplant* 19: 2107–2112
98 Chapman JR, Nankivell BJ (2006) Nephrotoxicity of ciclosporin A: short-term gain, long-term pain? *Nephrol Dial Transplant* 21: 2060–2063
99 Shihab FS, Bennett WM, Tanner AM, Andoh TF (1997) Angiotensin II blockade decreases TGF-β1 and matrix proteins in cyclosporine nephropathy. *Kidney Int* 52: 660–673
100 Islam M, Burke JF Jr, McGowan TA, Zhu Y, Dunn SR, McCue P, Kanalas J, Sharma K (2001) Effect of anti-transforming growth factor-beta antibodies in cyclosporine-induced renal dysfunction. *Kidney Int* 59: 498–506
101 Shihab FS, Yi H, Bennett WM, Andoh TF (2000) Effect of nitric oxide modulation on TGF-beta1 and matrix proteins in chronic cyclosporine nephrotoxicity. *Kidney Int* 58: 1174–1185
102 Pichler RH, Franceschini N, Young BA, Hugo C, Andoh TF, Burdmann EA, Shankland SJ, Alpers CE, Bennett WM, Couser WG (1995) Pathogenesis of cyclosporine nephropathy: Roles of angiotensin II and osteopontin. *J Am Soc Nephrol* 6: 1186–1196
103 Feutren G, Mihatsch MJ (1992) Risk factors for cyclosporine-induced nephropathy in patients with autoimmune diseases. International Kidney Biopsy Registry of Cyclosporine in Autoimmune Diseases. *N Engl J Med* 326: 1654–1660
104 Taler SJ, Textor SC, Canzanello VJ, Schwartz L (1999) Cyclosporin-induced hypertension. incidence, pathogenesis and management. *Drug Safety* 20: 437–449
105 Bennett WM, Porter GA (1988) Cyclosporin-associated hypertension. *Am J Med* 85: 131–133
106 Bennett WM (1997) Cyclosporine nephrotoxicity: implications for dermatology. *Int J Dermatol* 36: 11–14
107 Kamel KS, Ethier JH, Quaggin S, Levin A, Albert S, Carlisle EJ, Halperin ML (1992) Studies to determine the basis for hyperkalemia in recipients of a renal transplant who are treated with cyclosporine. *J Am Soc Nephrol* 2: 1279–1284
108 Ling BN, Eaton DC (1993) Cyclosporin A inhibits apical secretory K^+ channels in rabbit cortical collecting tubule principal cells. *Kidney Int* 44: 974–984

109 Barton CH, Vaziri ND, Martin DC, Choi S, Alikhani S (1987) Hypomagnesemia and renal magnesium wasting in renal transplant recipients receiving cyclosporine. *Am J Med* 83: 693–699
110 Schwartz RB, Bravo SM, Klufas RA, Hsu L, Barnes PD, Robson CD, Antin JH (1995) Cyclosporine neurotoxicity and its relationship to hypertensive encephalopathy: CT and MR findings in 16 cases. *AJR Am J Roentgenol* 165: 627–631
111 Hinchey J, Chaves C, Appignani B, Breen J, Pao L, Wang A, Pessin MS, Lamy C, Mas JL, Caplan LR (1996) A reversible posterior leukoencephalopathy syndrome. *N Engl J Med* 334: 494–500
112 Wijdicks EF, Wiesner RH, Krom RA (1995) Neurotoxicity in liver transplant recipients with cyclosporine immunosuppression. *Neurology* 45: 1962–1964
113 Marcil, I, Stern RS (2001) Squamous-cell cancer of the skin in patients given PUVA and ciclosporin: nested cohort crossover study. *Lancet* 358: 1042–1045
114 Paul CF, Ho VC, McGeown C, Christophers E, Schmidtmann B, Guillaume JC, Lamarque V, Dubertret L (2003) Risk of malignancies in psoriasis patients treated with cyclosporine: a 5 y cohort study. *J Invest Dermatol* 120: 211–216
115 HO VC (2004) The use of cyclosporin in psoriasis: a clinical review. *Br J Dermatol* 150: 1–10
116 Behnam SM, Behnam SE, Koo JY (2005) Review of cyclosporine immunosuppressive safety data in dermatology patients after two decades of use. *J Drugs Dermatol* 4: 189–194
117 Hojo M, Morimoto T, Maluccio M, Asano T, Morimoto K, Lagman M, Shimbo T, Suthanthiran M (1999) Cyclosporine induces cancer progression by a cell-autonomous mechanism. *Nature* 397: 530–534
118 Thomas DW, Newcombe RG, Osborne GR (2000) Risk factors in the development of cyclosporine-induced gingival overgrowth. *Transplantation* 69: 522–526
119 Wong W, Hodge MG, Lewis A, Sharpstone P, Kingswood JC (1994) Resolution of cyclosporin-induced gingival hypertrophy with metronidazole. *Lancet* 343: 986
120 Gomez E, Sanchez-Nunez M, Sanchez JE, Corte C, Aguado S, Portal C, Baltar J, Alvarez-Grande J (1997) Treatment of cyclosporin-induced gingival hyperplasia with azithromycin. *Nephrol Dial Transplant* 12: 2694–2697
121 Ishida Y, Matsuda H, Kida K (1995) Effect of cyclosporin A on human bone marrow granulocyte-macrophage progenitors with anti-cancer agents. *Acta Paediatr Jpn* 37: 610–613
122 van der Heide JJ, Bilo HJ, Donker JM, Wilmink JM, Tegzess AM (1993) Effect of dietary fish oil on renal function and rejection in cyclosporine-treated recipients of renal transplants. *N Engl J Med* 329: 769–773
123 Homan van der Heide JJ, Bilo HJ, Tegzess AM, Donker AJ (1990) The effects of dietary supplementation with fish oil on renal function in cyclosporine-treated renal transplant recipients. *Transplantation* 49: 523–527
124 Berthoux FC, Guerin C, Burgard G, Berthoux P, Alamartine E (1992) One-year randomized controlled trial with omega-3 fatty acid-fish oil in clinical renal transplantation. *Transplant Proc* 24: 2578–2582
125 Ruggenenti P, Perico N, Mosconi L, Gaspari F, Benigni A, Amuchastegui CS, Bruzzi I, Remuzzi G (1993) Calcium channel blockers protect transplant patients from cyclosporine-induced daily renal hypoperfusion. *Kidney Int* 43: 706–711
126 Rahn KH, Barenbrock M, Fritschka E, Heinecke A, Lippert J, Schroeder K, Hauser I, Wagner K, Neumayer HH (1999) Effect of nitrendipine on renal function in renal-transplant patients treated with cyclosporin: a randomised trial. *Lancet* 354: 1415–1420
127 Hunley TE, Fogo A, Iwasaki S, Kon V (1995) Endothelin A receptor mediates functional but not structural damage in chronic cyclosporine nephrotoxicity. *J Am Soc Nephrol* 5: 1718–1723
128 Burdmann EA, Andoh TF, Nast CC, Evan A, Connors BA, Coffman TM, Lindsley J, Bennett WM (1995) Prevention of experimental cyclosporine-induced interstitial fibrosis by losartan and enalapril. *Am J Physiol* 269: F491–499
129 Smith JR, Kubacki VB, Rakhit A, Martin LL, Schaffer AV, Jasani MK, Hefty DJ, Johnston T, Cannon C, Bennett WM (1993) Chronic thromboxane synthesis inhibition with CGS 12970 in human cyclosporine nephrotoxicity. *Transplantation* 56: 1422–1426
130 Lacour M, Mehta-Nikhad B, Atherton DJ, Harper JI (1996) An appraisal of acitretin therapy in children with inherited disorders of keratinization. *Br J Dermatol* 134: 1023–1029
131 Pereira TM, Vieira AP, Fernandes JC, Sousa-Basto A (2006) Cyclosporin A treatment in severe childhood posriasis. *J Eur Acad Dermatol Venereol* 20: 651–656
132 Berth-Jones H, Finlay AY, Zaki I, Tan B, Goodyear H, Lewis-Jones S, Cork MJ, Bleehen SS, Sale

MS, Allen BR et al. (1996) Cyclosporine in severe childhood atopic dermatitis: a multicenter study. *J Am Acad Dermatol* 34: 1016–1021
133 Harper JI, Berth-Jones J, Camp RD, Dillon MJ, Finlay AY, Holden CA, O'Sullivan D, Veys PA (2001) Cyclosporin for atopic dermatitis in children. *Dermatology* 203: 3–6
134 Robitaille P, Chartrand S, Stanley C, Chartrand C (1991) Long-term assessment of renal function under cyclosporine in pediatric heart transplant recipients. *J Heart Lung Transplant* 10: 460–463
135 Mahe E, Bodemer C, Pruszkowski A, Teillac-Hamel D, de Prost Y (2001) Cyclosporine in childhood psoriasis. *Arch Dermatol* 137: 1532–1533
136 Cooney GF, Habucky K, Hoppu K (1997) Cyclosporine pharmacokinetics in pediatric transplant recipients. *Clin Pharmacokinet* 32: 481–495
137 Nandakumaran M, Eldeen AS (1990) Transfer of cyclosporine in the perfused human placenta. *Dev Pharmacol Ther* 15: 101–105
138 Armenti VT, Ahiswede KM, Ahlsweded BA, Jarrell BE, Moritz MJ, Burke JF (1994) National transplantation pregnancy registry outcomes of 154 pregnancies in cyclosporine-treated female kidney transplant recipients. *Transplantation* 57: 502–506
139 Olshan AF, Mattison DR, Zwanenburg TS (1994) International Commission for Protection Against Environmental Mutagens and Carcinogens. Cyclosporine A: review of genotoxicity and potential for adverse human reproductive and developmental effects. Report of a Working Group on the genotoxicity of cyclosporine A, 18 August 1993. *Mutat Res* 317: 163–176
140 Petri M (2003) Immunosuppressive drug use in pregnancy. *Autoimmunity* 36: 51–56
141 Griffiths CEM, Clark CM, Chalmers RJG, Li Wan PO A, Williams HC (2000) A systematic review of treatments for severe psoriasis. *Health Technol Assess* 4: 1–125
142 Naldi L, Griffiths CEM (2005) Traditional therapies in the management of moderate to severe chronic plaque psoriasis: an assessment of the benefits and risks. *Br J Dermatol* 152: 597–615
143 Griffiths CEM, Dubertret L, Ellis CN, Finlay AY, Finzi AF, Ho VC, Johnston A, Katsambas A, Lison AE, Naeyaert HM et al. (2004) Ciclosporin in psoriasis clinical practice: an international consensus statement. *Br J Dermatol* 150: 11–23
144 Heydendael VM, Spuls PI, Opmeer BC, de Borgie CA, Reitsma JB, Goldschmidt WF, Bossuyt PM, Bos JD, de Rie MA (2003) Methotrexate *versus* cyclosporine in moderate-to-severe chronic plaque psoriasis. *N Engl J Med* 349: 658–665

Treatment of Psoriasis
Edited by J.M. Weinberg

Traditional systemic therapy II: retinoids and others (hydroxyurea, thiopurine antimetabolites, mycophenlic acid, sulfasalazine)

Sejal K. Shah and Jeffrey M. Weinberg

St. Luke's-Roosevelt Hospital Center, Department of Dermatology, 1090 Amsterdam Avenue, Suite 11D, New York, NY 10025, USA

Many systemic agents are commonly used to treat generalized psoriasis. Although they are efficacious, their potential adverse effects require close monitoring. These agents can be used either alone or in combination therapy. In addition, they can be used as rotational or sequential therapies.

Retinoids

The oral retinoids are vitamin A metabolites that were introduced for clinical use in the 1970s and have since been established as a successful treatment for psoriasis. Initially found to be useful anticancer agents, they were subsequently studied in proliferative disorders because of their effects on proliferation, differentiation and apoptosis. Although the exact pathogenesis of psoriasis is unknown, an abnormal vitamin A metabolism may play a role.

Retinol, the natural form of vitamin A, is converted to the active form, all-trans-retinoic acid (ATRA), through the sequential enzymatic activity of retinol dehydrogenase and retinal dehydrogenase (Fig. 1). A binding protein, cellular retinol binding protein-1 (CRBP 1), acts as a cofactor in the reactions. Cellular retinoic acid binding proteins 1 and 2 (CRABP 1 and CRABP 2) balance the levels of free ATRA in the cell and facilitate its metabolism [1]. ATRA binds nuclear retinoic acid receptors (RARs) to produce cellular effects; 9-cis-retinoic acid binds both nuclear retinoid X receptors (RXRs) as well as RARs. ATRA is metabolized by cytochrome P450 enzymes in the CYP 26 family [2, 3].

Compared to normal skin, psoriatic skin has been found to have increased rates of ATRA production and levels of CRABP 2 with no significant difference in receptor levels [3]. As Th-1 type cytokine activity mediates psoriasis, the increased ATRA production is likely a secondary event. Interferonβ, a Th-1 cytokine that is increased in psoriatic skin, has been shown to elevate retinoic acid levels [4]. Acitretin may exert its efficacy by (1) blocking the cytokine-induced retinoic acid production and affecting cytokine expression, (2)

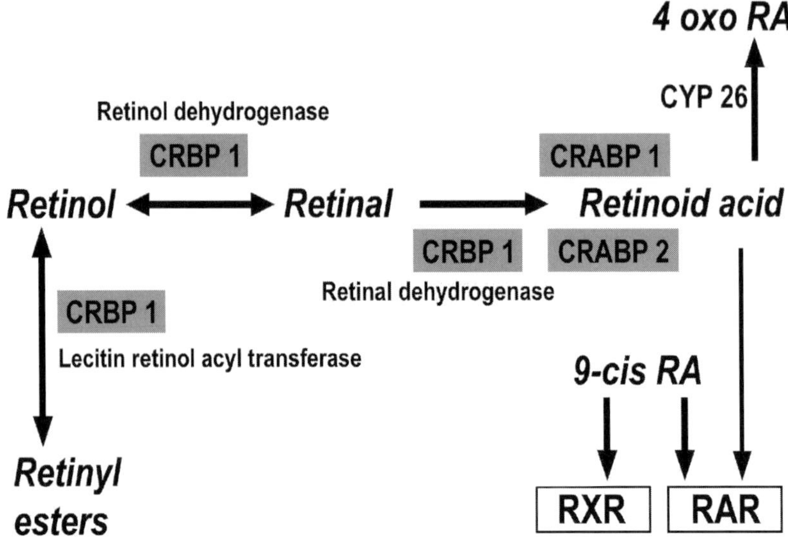

Figure 1. Cellular retinoid pathway. RA: Retinoic Acid; CRABP: Cellular Retinoic Acid Binding Protein; CRBP: Cellular Retinol Binding Protein; CYP: Cytochrome P450 enzyme; RAR: nuclear Retinoic Acid Receptor; RXR: nuclear Retinoid X Receptor. Reprinted from *J Am Acad Dermatol*, Volume 41, Saurat JH, Retinoids and psoriasis: Novel issues in retinoid pharmacology and implications for psoriasis treatment, Page S3, Copyright 1999, with permission from The American Academy of Dermatology, Inc.

increasing CRABP 2 levels thereby promoting ATRA metabolism, or (3) altering CYP 26 enzyme activity [3].

Etretinate, the first systemic retinoid approved for psoriasis, was removed from the market in 1998 due to safety concerns related to its lipophilic nature. Acitretin, the primary active metabolite of etretinate, was introduced in the late 1980s. Because acitretin is significantly less lipophilic than etretinate, it is not as readily stored in the body and is completely eliminated from the body within 2 months compared to at least 2 years for etretinate. Currently, acitretin is the only oral retinoid approved for the treatment of psoriasis.

Acitretin is primarily effective in the treatment of pustular and erythrodermic psoriasis. For guttate and plaque psoriasis, it is more successful when combined with other therapies [5, 6].

Double-blind, controlled trials comparing acitretin (Soriatane) to placebo have found acitretin to be an efficacious therapy for psoriasis. Patients with severe psoriasis covering at least 10% body surface area were treated with daily Soriatane, either 25 mg (74 patients) or 50 mg (100 patients), or placebo (101 patients). After 8 weeks of treatment, all 174 patients in the treatment group had a statistically significant improvement (p-value < 0.05) in regards to physician's global evaluation, erythema, scale, and thickness when compared to baseline and placebo. Continued improvement was noted in patients who received treatment for a total of 6 months, 12 months and 18 months [7]. An evaluation of 12 clinical trials in which 25–35 mg of acitretin daily was used to treat various dermatoses found that 31.5% of psoriasis patients achieved complete remission and 46.5% experienced marked improvement. 8.5% had no improvement or worsening of their psoriasis. Authors further analyzed results by subtype and noted that 100% of pustular-type and 83.3% of erythrodermic-type responded completely or markedly compared to 76.5% of other types (primarily plaque-type) [8].

As monotherapy, acitretin is most effective in a dose range of 25–50 mg daily (Tab. 1). Response is gradual, and patients may initially worsen before improving. Generally, 3–6 months are required to achieve a maximal response. Dose escalation has been recommended as a useful approach to determine the safest and most effective dose for a patient, especially when acitretin is part of a combination therapy. Treatment is started at low doses (10–25 mg daily) and escalated as needed to maximize efficacy and minimize adverse effects [6]. A complete blood cell count (CBC), complete metabolic profile (CMP), pregnancy test, fasting lipid profile and urinalysis should be checked before initiating treatment. CBC, renal function, and urinalysis should be monitored every 3 months; a pregnancy test should be repeated monthly or as clinically indicated [9, 10]. Liver function tests and fasting lipid profile should be repeated every 1 to 2 weeks until stable, then as clinically indicated or every 3 months [7, 9]. Laboratory testing should be performed more frequently as clinically indicated [11, 12]. Acitretin should be taken with food to be adequately absorbed [12, 13].

Table 1. How to prescribe acitretin

1. Check baseline CBC, CMP, fasting lipid profile, pregnancy test, and urinalysis
2. Initiate therapy at 25–50 mg/day, maintenance therapy 25–50 mg/day
3. Repeat fasting lipid profile and liver function tests (LFTs) every 1–2 weeks until stable, then as clinically indicated or every 3 months
4. Repeat CBC, renal function tests, urinalysis every 3 months
5. Repeat pregnancy test every month or as clinically indicated
6. Hold if LFTs three times above upper limit of normal, triglycerides exceed 400 mg/dl, visual difficulties, or pregnancy

Adverse effects of retinoids

Several potential adverse effects have been associated with acitretin; however, they can be minimized by judicious patient selection and close monitoring. Acitretin is FDA pregnancy category X and should not be prescribed to women who are pregnant or nursing. Furthermore, it should not be given to women who are considering a pregnancy during treatment or for up to 3 years after treatment. All women of reproductive potential should start using contraception 1 month before beginning therapy and continue use for 3 years after therapy. A 3-year contraceptive period after therapy is recommended because when combined with ethanol, acitretin may be re-esterified into etretinate, which requires at least 2 years to be completely eliminated from the body. Therefore, female patients of child-bearing potential should be advised to abstain from alcohol during treatment and for 2 months after treatment [7]. The teratogenic potential of acitretin treatment in a male at the time of conception is unknown. For that reason, it is recommended that men receiving acitretin should use condoms during the treatment period and for 1 month after completing treatment [14, 15].

Toxicity to both the liver and pancreas has been associated with acitretin use. Increases in liver enzymes occur in approximately one third of patients; however, they are usually transient and reversible when the dose is reduced or treatment is stopped [7]. In an open-label study of 128 patients in which 87 patients underwent liver biopsies before and after acitretin treatment, liver pathology improved or did not change in 83% of patients [7]. Another report showed evidence of hepatitis in only 0.26% of 1'877 patients receiving acitretin [12, 16]. The most common lab abnormality that occurs with acitretin therapy is hyperlipidemia, especially hypertriglyceridemia [15]. Rare cases of pancreatitis, including fatal fulminant pancreatitis, have been reported [7]. In addition, patients may be at an increased risk for cardiovascular complications; both myocardial infarctions and thromboembolic events have been reported [7]. Patients may require lipid reduction through lifestyle modification, lipid-lowering medications, or dose reduction. Treatment should be discontinued if triglyceride levels reach above 400 mg/dL [15, 17].

Pseudotumor cerebri has been reported with systemic retinoid use but more commonly occurs with concurrent tetracycline antibiotic use [7, 10]. Patients who complain of headaches, visual changes, nausea or vomiting should be evaluated for papilledema, and pseudotumor cerebri should be ruled out. Dose-related mucocutaneous effects, such as cheilitis, alopecia, conjunctivitis, dry eyes, dry or peeling skin, and nail plate abnormalities commonly occur and are treated symptomatically [12]. Retinoid use may also be associated with hyperostosis and extra-skeletal calcification, which may cause pain, difficulty moving, or neurologic symptoms [7, 10, 12, 18].

Hydroxyurea

Hydroxyurea was introduced as an antineoplastic agent in 1960. It is primarily used in the management of hematological and neoplastic disorders. Its success in the treatment of recalcitrant psoriasis was first reported in 1969; a subsequent double-blind study by Leavell and Yarbro confirmed hydroxyurea's efficacy [19, 20].

There are several hypotheses regarding hydroxyurea's mechanism of action. Hydroxyurea inhibits ribonucleotide reductase, which catalyzes the conversion of ribonucleotides to deoxyribonucleotides, the rate-limiting step in DNA synthesis. DNA production is impaired at the S-phase of the cell cycle thereby inhibiting DNA replication; cells in the G1/S-phase accumulate and eventually undergo apoptosis [21]. It also affects pyrimidine synthesis and blocks pyrimidine nucleoside incorporation into DNA [22–24]. In the basal layer of the epidermis, hydroxyurea has been noted to inhibit cell replication [21, 24–26]. It has been shown alter neutrophil counts and chemotaxis [24, 27–28]. Lastly, hydroxyurea has been noted to normalize the amount of keratin in psoriatic plaques [20].

Most studies have focused on the hydroxyurea's role in the treatment of plaque-type psoriasis. Variable results have been reported when using it for the treatment of pustular psoriasis [24, 27, 29]. Guttate and erythrodermic forms have also been shown to respond to hydroxyurea [29].

Leavell and Yarbro conducted the first published double-blind study to evaluate the efficacy of hydroxyurea in the treatment of psoriasis. In their 8-week study, subjects were given placebo for 4 weeks and 1 g daily of hydroxyurea for 4 weeks in random order. 9 out of 10 patients improved clinically and histologically with hydroxyurea therapy [20]. Layton et al. treated 85 patients with widespread chronic plaque psoriasis, previously resistant to conventional topical therapy, with hydroxyurea therapy. Prior systemic therapy had not been used by any of the patients. Hydroxyurea was initiated at a dose of 1.5 g daily and adjusted based on clinical response and adverse effects. Most patients were maintained on 0.5–1.5 g per day with an average treatment length of 16 months (range 3–96 months). In cases of full remission, the dose was decreased slowly and discontinued if possible. The researchers reported a complete to near complete response in 51 patients (60%) and moderate clearing in 17 patients (20%) [30]. In a later study by Kumar et al., 31 Indian patients with extensive chronic plaque psoriasis (at least 20% body surface area) were treated with 1–1.5 g of hydroxyurea daily for an average of 36 weeks (range 6–136 weeks). The Psoriasis Area and Severity Index (PASI) score was used to rate response to treatment. 8 patients (26%) experienced a complete or near complete response, defined as a decrease in PASI score of at least 90%. A good response, a reduction in PASI score of 70–90%, was observed in 17 patients (55%) [31].

Hydroxyurea is readily absorbed after oral administration. It is excreted by the kidneys and serum levels are undetectable within 24 h [24]. Therapy is usually initiated at 1 g per day and increased monthly by increments of 500 mg per day if needed (Tab. 2). Dosing ranges from 1–2 g daily in divided doses of 500 mg. A complete blood count (CBC), complete metabolic panel (CMP), and urinalysis should be checked before starting treatment. While on hydroxyurea, CBC should be repeated weekly for the first 4 weeks, then every 2–4 weeks. Liver function tests and urinalysis should be repeated monthly [9, 24, 32].

Table 2. How to prescribe hydroxyurea

1. Check baseline CBC, CMP, and urinalysis
2. Initiate treatment at 1 gm/day
3. Adjust dose monthly by increments of 500 mg/day
4. Repeat CBC weekly for the first 4 weeks of treatment, then every 2–4 weeks
5. Repeat LFTs and urinalysis monthly
6. Hold if severe anemia, white blood cell count (WBC) is <2'500/μL or platelet count is <100'000/μL

Adverse effects of hydroxyurea

In most studies, hydroxyurea appears to be relatively well-tolerated. Leavell and Yarbro did not report any toxic effects in their study subjects [20]; Layton et al. reported adverse effects in 43% (37/85) of patients and 18% (16/85) of patients were required to stop treatment due to a side effect [30]. While Kumar et al. reported adverse effects, no patients required treatment cessation [31]. However, there are safety concerns, specifically related to hydroxyurea's effect on the bone marrow. One author reported that almost 50% of patients who improve significantly with hydroxyurea experience bone marrow toxicity [10]. In one study the majority of side effects noted were hematological and included anemia (11.7%), leukopenia (7%), thrombocytopenia (2.3%), and pancytopenia (11.7%). In most cases, the blood counts normalized after discontinuing treatment or lowering the dose [30]. A reversible macrocytosis occurs in almost all patients treated with hydroxyurea but rarely requires treatment or cessation of hydroxyurea [10, 30, 31].

Hydroxyurea is also known to have several mucocutaneous effects. The incidence of these types of reactions has varied greatly among studies. In one study of only Indian patients, mucocutaneous reactions developed in 64.5% (20/31) of the patients after an average of 6.3 weeks of therapy [31]. In a related report, mucocutaneous effects were observed in 65.5% (19/29) of the patients treated, most commonly grayish-brown pigmentation of the skin, nails, or mucosa. Researchers noted that there may be a racial predisposition for these types of reactions [33]. Other dermatological effects that have been reported include actinic psoriasis, alopecia, lower extremity edema, leg ulcers, oral ulcers, xerosis, dermatomyositis-like poikiloderma, burning sensation at sites of lesions, palpable purpura, cutaneous vasculitis, fixed drug eruption, actinic keratoses, and squamous cell carcinoma [29, 31, 33].

Some studies have reported an increase in liver enzymes and a mild hepatitis; irreversible liver damage has not been documented [24, 30, 34–37]. Patients may also experience nausea, vomiting, anorexia or dyspepsia [30, 32]. Renal dysfunction has been reported [24, 32, 38]. Hydroxyurea is FDA pregnancy category D. Both male and female patients should be advised appropriately. In addition, women who are nursing should not receive the drug [32].

Thiopurine antimetabolites

The thiopurine antimetabolites are steroid-sparing immunosuppressants and include azathioprine (AZA), 6-mercaptopurine (6-MP), and 6-thioguanine (6-TG). AZA, which was initially used in renal transplant patients, is a synthetic purine analog that is rapidly converted to 6-MP by a nonenzymatic process. 6-MP is then metabolized by one of three competing enzymes; thiopurine methyltransferase (TPMT), xanthine oxidase (XO), or hypoxanthine-guanine phosphoribosyl transferase (HGPRT) (Fig. 2). Only HGPRT converts 6-MP to active 6-thioguanine metabolites [39]. The active 6-TG metabolites act at the S-phase of the cell cycle to inhibit *de novo* synthesis of purine bases, which T- and B-lymphocytes depend upon. In addition, effects on natural killer cell (NKC) function, T cell signaling and cytotoxic activity, prostaglandin production, and neutrophil trafficking has been reported [40].

XO converts only 6-MP into inactive metabolites by catalyzing its oxidation; whereas TPMT catalyzes the S-methylation of both 6-MP and 6-TG to

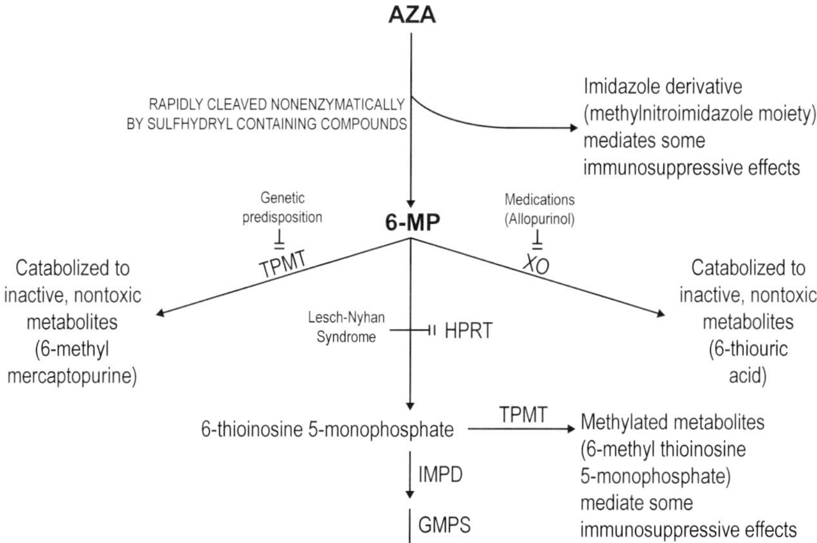

Figure 2. Azathioprine metabolism. TPMT: Thiopurine Methyltransferase; XO: Xanthine Oxidase; HPRT: Hypoxanthine-Guanine Phosphoribosyl Transferase. Reprinted from *J Am Acad Dermatol*, Volume 55, Patel AA, Swerlick RA, McCall CO, Azathioprine in dermatology: The past, the present, and the future, Page 371, Copyright 2006, with permission from The American Academy of Dermatology, Inc.

yield inactive metabolites [39]. In humans, TPMT activity is controlled by a genetic polymorphism. Homozygotes for the low activity allele have minimal or absent TPMT activity and are at risk for severe myelosuppression when treated with thiopurine antimetabolites [39]. Heterozygotes display intermediate enzyme activity, which can vary greatly, and usually develop a mild to moderate myelosuppression when treated with thiopurine antimetabolites [41, 42]. Individuals with elevated enzyme activity may not respond therapeutically to thiopurine medications. In a retrospective analysis of 3'291 patients who had undergone testing for TPMT activity, 80% of the patients exhibited normal activity, 9% higher than normal activity, and 10% low activity [43]. 0.45% of the study population was found to have undetectable activity which is higher than the previously reported frequency of 0.3% [43, 44]. Because TPMT may be inducible, the researchers also analyzed the results of the individuals in whom TPMT was measured before the initiation treatment and found the same distribution in those 1'747 patients [43]. Due to this variability, testing for TPMT activity levels appears to be valuable and cost-effective [42]. Enzyme activity can be measured by a radiochemical functional assay using red blood cells or nonradioactive high-performance liquid chromatography (HPLC). Genotyping is also available; however, it may not be as cost-effective because of the existence of multiple mutant alleles [42, 43].

Du Vivier et al. used azathioprine to treat 29 patients with severe plaque type psoriasis, pustular psoriasis, and erythrodermic psoriasis. 66% (19/29) of the patients showed an improvement of 50–100% on doses of 75–200 mg/day [45]. Zackheim et al. retrospectively studied 76 patients with plaque-type psoriasis and five patients with palmoplantar pustular psoriasis treated with 6-TG. Patients with rapidly progressive disease were dosed daily and most were maintained on 80–160 mg of 6-TG daily. Patients with stable but resistant disease were dosed twice a week and maintained on 120–240 mg twice a week. 37 of the 76 patients (48.8%) with plaque-type psoriasis were 'effectively' maintained on 6-TG therapy for median of 33 months (range 3–145 months). The remainder of the patients discontinued treatment due to initial treatment failure (4 patients, 5.3%), relapse while on treatment (8 patients, 10.5%) or adverse effects (27 patients, 35.5%). Four of the five patients with palmoplantar pustular psoriasis were 'effectively' maintained for 4–36 months [46]. In another study, 17 of 18 (94%) patients treated for at least 8 weeks improved by at least 50% on an average dose of 50 mg of 6-TG daily (range 40 mg weekly–120 mg daily). Of note, subjects were not required to discontinue adjunctive therapies, including phototherapy, topical treatments, and other systemic treatments [47].

Azathioprine is well-absorbed from the digestive tract and does not cross the blood-brain barrier. The recommended daily dose for dermatological diseases is 1–3 mg/kg [48]. TPMT levels, as well as a CBC, CMP, and urinalysis, should be checked at baseline. It should not be prescribed to individuals with very low or no TPMT activity. Patients with low activity should be treated with 0.5–1 mg/kg/day and closely monitored for myelotoxicity; patients with normal or high TPMT activity can be treated with 1–3 mg/kg/day [42, 48]. Treatment is usually initiated at 50 mg daily and increased by 50 mg increments every 4 weeks until clinical response, toxicity, or a maximum dose of 300 mg/day (Tab. 3) [9]. Generally, if no response is seen after 3 months, it should be discontinued. A trial dosage above the recommended maximum dose may be considered in patients who fail to respond and do not experience adverse effects or who have high TPMT activity [48]. CBC and CMP should be repeated every 4 weeks during dose escalation, then every 3 months when the maintenance dose is achieved. If liver function tests are elevated, pancreatic enzymes should be checked [9].

6-TG is incompletely and variably absorbed after oral administration, on average 30% is absorbed (range 14–46%) [49]. Baseline laboratory testing and monitoring of liver and kidney function (CMP) is similar to that for azathioprine. However, as it is more likely to cause bone marrow suppression, CBC should be performed at baseline and monitored weekly during the dose escalation period, then every 2 weeks [9]. Generally, dosing is initiated at 20 mg daily and increased by 20 mg increments every 2 weeks up to 80–120 mg daily until clinical response or toxicity occur (Tab. 4) [21]. After desirable clinical response is achieved, tapering the dose to twice or three times weekly can be

Table 3. How to prescribe azathioprine

1. Check baseline CBC, CMP, TPMT, urinalysis
2. Initiate treatment at 50 mg/day
3. Dose can be increased by increments of 50 mg/day every 4 weeks
4. Repeat CBC and CMP monthly during dose escalation, then every 3 months once maintenance reached
5. If LFTs are elevated check pancreatic enzymes
6. Maximum daily dose is 300 mg/day
7. Hold if severe gastrointestinal symptoms, signs of anemia, leucopenia, or thrombocytopenia on CBC

Table 4. How to prescribe 6-thioguanine

1. Check baseline CBC, CMP, TPMT, urinalysis
2. Initiate treatment at 20 mg/day or 80–120 mg twice a week
3. Dose can be increased by increments of 20 mg/day every 2 weeks or by 20 mg/2–3 times a week every 2–4 weeks
4. Repeat CMP monthly during dose escalation then every 3 months once maintenance reached
5. Repeat CBC weekly during dose escalation, then every 2 weeks
6. Hold if WBC < 4'000/μL, platelet count < 125'000/μL, or hemoglobin < 11 gm/dL or at first sign of large decrease in blood count on CBC

attempted [9]. Alternatively, pulse dosing has also been recommended. Treatment is initiated at 80–100 mg of 6-TG twice a week and increased by 20 mg increments every 2–4 weeks until clinical response or toxicity. The maximum dose is 480 mg per week [46, 50].

Adverse effects of thiopurine antimetabolites

Azathioprine appears to be well-tolerated. Gastrointestinal adverse effects are most commonly associated with its use and include nausea, vomiting, or diarrhea. The symptoms may mimic a viral gastroenteritis. These effects are rarely severe enough to require treatment cessation and can usually be managed by reducing or dividing the dose or taking it with food [42, 45]. If, however, the symptoms are severe, the patient may be developing a potentially fatal hypersensitivity reaction and treatment should be stopped immediately. Hypersensitivity reactions usually occur in the first month of treatment. They can present with a variety of symptoms, including fever, hypotension, shock, acute renal failure, rhabdomyolysis, vasculitis, urticaria, maculopapular rash, arthralgias and myalgias [40, 42, 51]. Hepatotoxicity, hepatic veno-occlusive disease and pancreatitis have been associated with its use but are uncommon and more likely in patients with underlying gastrointestinal diseases [42]. Du Vivier et al. did not report any liver function abnormalities or severe liver damage on biopsy, only reversible mild portal fibrosis and cholestasis were observed [45].

Bone marrow suppression is also a well-known effect of azathioprine [21, 40, 42]. It can manifest as leukopenia, anemia, thrombocytopenia, or pancytopenia; and may be severe. du Vivier et al. observed a reversible leukopenia in 10 of 29 subjects. All subjects recovered with either dosage reduction or temporary treatment cessation. Anemia, which responded to iron therapy and dose reduction, was noted in one subject. Thrombocytopenia, requiring discontinuation of azathioprine, was noted in another. Macrocytosis was also reported in 12 of 29 patients [45].

Dermatologic effects such as alopecia, allergic contact dermatitis, hyperpigmentation, verrucae, herpes zoster, dermatomycoses and Norwegian scabies have been reported with azathioprine use [42]. Patients may have an increased risk of developing infections and malignancies secondary to immunosuppression [40, 42]

The side effect profile for 6-TG is similar to that of azathioprine; however, bone marrow toxicity seems to occur more commonly. Both Zackheim et al. and Mason and Krueger reported it as the most common adverse effect in their subjects [46, 47]. In the study by Zackheim et al., 46.9% (38/81) of patients developed myelosuppression, most frequently leukopenia (42%; 34/81 patients). Anemia was observed in 11.1% (9/81) of patients and thrombocytopenia in 8.6% (7/81). 21% (17/81) of patients were required to stop treatment secondary to bone marrow suppression [46].

Elevations in liver enzymes also appear to occur more commonly with 6-TG therapy. Of the 60 patients who had liver function tested in the study published by Zackheim et al., 15 (25%) had an increase in levels; these abnormalities led to the cessation of treatment in six patients (10%). One patient experienced acute hepatitis, but fully recovered after stopping 6-TG [46]. Hepatic veno-occlusive disease has also been reported with its use [10, 49, 52].

Other reported side effects include nausea, vomiting, diarrhea, oral aphthous ulcers, gastric ulcers, gastroesophageal reflux, fatigue, headaches, myalgias, and joint stiffness [46, 47, 49]. Dermatologic effects include herpes zoster, verrucae vulgaris, drug eruption, photodermatitis, and pruritis [46, 47]. Zackheim et al. reported the development of multiple skin cancers, squamous cell and basal cell, in four patients. Skin cancers were observed in both sun-exposed and non-exposed areas [46].

In general, the severity of the adverse effect is inversely related to the TPMT activity level, and more severe effects are more likely to occur in patients with low or absent TPMT activity. Additionally, allopurinol, an XO inhibitor, may increase toxicity by decreasing the production of inactive metabolites. Benzoic acid derivatives, such as sulfasalazine, may inhibit TPMT thereby increasing active metabolites and toxicity [40, 42].

Both azathioprine and 6-TG are FDA pregnancy category D. The fetus may be protected from toxicity because the immature liver is unable to convert 6-MP into active metabolites [42]. Several reports have documented normal infants without congenital abnormalities born to mothers taking these medications for other conditions [42, 53, 54]. These medications should not be prescribed to nursing women because of the potential risk of immunosuppression and carcinogenesis, which outweigh the benefits of nursing [42]. Studies have also suggested that the use of thiopurine antimetabolites in males before conception may impose a risk to the fetus [55, 56].

Mycophenolic acid

The immunosuppressant mycophenolic acid (MPA) is a reversible and non-competitive inhibitor of inosine monophosphate dehydrogenase. It therefore blocks *de novo* purine synthesis and DNA and RNA production, which affects T- and B-lymphocyte proliferation and subsequently antibody production [21, 40, 57, 58]. MPA was first used successfully to treat psoriasis in the 1970s [10]. The prodrug mycophenolate mofetil (MMF), a morpholinoethyl ester of MPA, was introduced in the 1990s. MMF is converted to MPA via ester hydrolysis in the liver [40]. The liver further metabolizes MPA into its inactive glucuronide. Certain cell types, such as human epidermal cells and those that line the gastrointestinal tract, contain an abundance of β-Glucuronidase, which converts the inactive form back into active MPA [59].

Jones et al. published the first study documenting the efficacy of MPA in treating psoriasis. In this pilot study, 29 patients with psoriasis were treated with a median daily dose of 3'600 mg (range 2'400–4'800 mg/day) for at least 12 weeks. Authors noted complete clearing in one patient, almost complete clearing in 14 patients, definite improvement in 13, and minimal improvement in one. The baseline mean severity score was 47 (range 21–88); after the 12-week treatment period, it was 15 (range 0–50), which was a decrease of 68% [60]. Subsequent studies confirmed these results [61–64]. Haufs et al. reported the first case of psoriasis successfully treated with MMF [65]. Geilen et al. treated 11 patients with severe stable plaque psoriasis with MMF for a total of 6 weeks. Patients received 1 g twice a day for the first 3 weeks followed by 500 mg twice a day for the remaining 3 weeks. The PASI was used to evaluate response to treatment; the baseline mean PASI score was 30.5 (range 12–53). During the first half of the study, the PASI score decreased by 40–70% in seven patients, by 25–39% in three patients, and by less than 25% in one patient. At end of the 6-week study period, the mean PASI score was 16.1, which was a reduction of 47% [58]. A subsequent 12-week, open-label trial completed by 18 patients with moderate to severe psoriasis who were treated with up to 3 g daily of MMF (2 gm per day for 2 weeks then 3 gm per day for 10 weeks) found MMF to be an effective monotherapy. At week 12, the PASI score had decreased by at least 37% (range 37–98%) in 14 patients (77%), with 11 patients (61%) experiencing a reduction of at least 50%. Four patients (22%) had little or no response to MMF treatment [66].

After oral administration, MMF is rapidly and almost completely absorbed. Once absorbed, it undergoes rapid conversion to MPA. The majority (87%) of the drug is excreted in the urine as MPA glucuronide [67]. A baseline CBC, CMP, urinalysis, and pregnancy test should be checked. Dosing is usually initiated at 500 mg four times a day and adjusted by 250 mg a day every 4 weeks based on clinical response and dose-limiting toxicity (Tab. 5). The maximum daily dose is 4 g daily. CBC should be monitored weekly for the first month, then every 2 weeks for the next month, then monthly [10]. CMP and other testing should be repeated every 3 months or as clinically indicated [9].

Table 5. How to prescribe mycophenolate mofetil

1. Check baseline CBC, CMP, urinalysis, and pregnancy test
2. Initiate treatment at 500 mg four times a day
3. Adjust dose by increments of 250 mg/day every 4 weeks
4. Repeat CBC weekly for the first month of treatment, then every 2 weeks for the second month, then monthly
5. Repeat other testing every 3 months or as clinically indicated
6. Maximum dose is 4 gm/day

Adverse effects of mycophenolic acid

Gastrointestinal adverse effects are the most common toxicity associated with MPA and MMF use. Nausea, vomiting, diarrhea, abdominal cramps, constipation, and bloody stools have been reported [40, 59, 61, 62, 67, 68]. These adverse effects are generally dose-related, rarely severe, and usually minimized by reducing or dividing the dose [21, 40, 59, 61]. A significant toxicity to the liver has not been documented. Zhou et al. noted that five patients developed transient mild gastrointestinal symptoms that did not require any changes in treatment [66]. Geilen et al. did not report any gastrointestinal adverse effects [58].

MPA and MMF may affect the hematopoietic system; anemia, thrombocytopenia, and leukopenia can occur. These effects are generally dose-related and reversible when the dose is lowered or discontinued [21, 59, 60, 62, 66]. An increased risk of bacterial and viral infections has been associated with MMF and MPA use and is likely secondary to immunosuppression. In most cases, they are uncomplicated; and after resolution patients are able to resume treatment without recurrence. Infectious complications reported with MPA use include herpes zoster, herpes simplex, verruca vulgaris, condyloma acuminata, upper respiratory infections, flu-like syndrome, pharyngitis, bronchitis, gastroenteritis, and urinary tract infections [61, 62, 64]. An increased frequency of herpetic viral infections has been noted in several studies [61, 62, 64]. An increased incidence of infections with MMF treatment has been primarily shown in transplant patient and has not been reported in psoriatic patients treated with MMF [40, 59].

Patients may also be at an increased risk for malignancy [61, 64, 67]. Epinette et al. reported malignancies in six patients. Two patients developed uncomplicated basal cell carcinomas. The other four patients developed noncutaneous malignancies; however, the authors noted that the study incidence of these cancers did not differ significantly from the incidence of cancer for a similar population in the US [64]. In randomized, controlled, double-blind trials of kidney transplant patients receiving MPA (Myfortic), the incidence of malignancy is consistent with that previously reported for this population [68]. In renal transplant patients receiving MMF, the incidence of lymphoproliferative malignancies is 1–2% and up to 5.5% for other noncutaneous malignancies [10, 69]. Studies of 1'483 renal transplant patients treated with MMF (CellCept) for prevention of graft rejection found the incidence of malignancy to be similar to that reported previously in the literature for renal transplant patients. In trials of renal, cardiac and hepatic transplant patients treated with 2–3 g daily of MMF (CellCept) with other immunosuppressants, 0.4–1% of patients developed lymphoproliferative diseases, 1.6–4.2% developed nonmelanoma skin cancers, and 0.7–2.1% developed other types of cancers. The incidence did not change unpredictably in the 3-year data when compared to the 1-year data [67]. Malignancies have not been reported in psoriasis patients treated with MMF [58, 65, 66].

Genitourinary symptoms including dysuria, frequency, urgency, vaginal bleeding or burning, and sterile pyuria may occur [61, 64, 67, 68]. A significant renal toxicity has not been reported [59, 62, 70–72]. Neurologic effects such as weakness, fatigue, insomnia, tinnitus and headache have been reported [61, 62, 64, 67, 68]. MMF and MPA are FDA pregnancy category C.

Sulfasalazine

Sulfasalazine is a prodrug that is cleaved into 5-aminosalicylic acid (5-ASA; mesalamine) and sulfapyridine by bacteria in the colon. The exact mechanism of action of sulfasalazine is not fully understood; however several theories have been investigated. Studies have shown that it may prevent T- and B-lymphocyte proliferation by inhibiting DNA synthesis. It may also act as an anti-inflammatory by preventing the production of inflammatory leukotrienes, prostaglandins, and cytokines as well as impeding the function of macrophages and neutrophils (phagocytosis, chemotaxis, and adhesion) [73]. In psoriatic skin, arachidonic acid levels are increased, as are 5-lipoxygenase and 12-lipoxygenase activity. There is a resultant increase in the production of leukotrienes and a subsequent increase in inflammation [74]. Sulfasalazine likely exerts its therapeutic effect in psoriasis by inhibiting the 5-lipoxygenase pathway [74, 75]. In published trials, sulfasalazine has primarily been studied as a therapy for psoriatic arthritis, but has been shown to be effective in treating pustular and plaque-type psoriasis, as well [74–77].

Gupta et al. conducted an open-label trial in which 24 patients were treated with 1 g of sulfasalazine three times a day for 8 weeks. Two (8%) patients were clear at the end of the study. 10 (42%) patients experienced an improvement of 50–90%; and improvement of 25–50% was observed in seven (29%) patients [75]. A subsequent double-blind study in which 50 patients with moderate-to-severe plaque psoriasis were treated with either 3–4 g daily of sulfasalazine (23 patients) or placebo (27 patients) for 6–8 weeks also found sulfasalazine to be a successful therapeutic option. Of the 17 patients in the treatment group that completed the study, 14 patients (82%) had an improvement of at least 30%. In the placebo group, the majority (81%) of the patients had minimal-to-no response (less that 29% improvement), and four (15%) patients experienced an exacerbation. Compared to the placebo group, the sulfasalazine group improved significantly (p-value < 0.0001) in regards to global severity, erythema, scale, thickness, and total body surface area. Continued improvement was observed in the 14 patients in the treatment group received an additional 4 weeks of treatment [74].

Less than 15% of orally administered sulfasalazine is absorbed; however, in the intestine, bacteria metabolize it into sulfapyridine (SP) and 5-amiosalicylic acid (5-ASA) which are both well-absorbed from the intestine. Baseline CBC, CMP, and urinalysis should be checked before starting therapy [78]. Therapy is should be initiated at 500 mg three times a day. If this dose is tolerated for 3 days, it can be increased to 1 g three times a day (Tab. 6). After 6 weeks, the dose can be increased to 1 g four times a day if tolerated by the patient. Clinical efficacy should be noticeable by 4–6 weeks [74]. Laboratory testing should be monitored every 2 weeks during the first 3 months, then monthly during the next 3 months, then every 3 months or as clinically indicated [10, 78].

Table 6. How to prescribe sulfasalazine

1. Check baseline CBC, CMP, and urinalysis
2. Initiate treatment at 500 mg three times a day; if tolerated, increase to 1 gm three times a day
3. After 6 weeks, dose can be increased to 1 gm four times a day
4. Repeat laboratory testing every 2 weeks during the first 3 months, then monthly during the next 3 months, then every 3 months or as clinically indicated

Adverse effects of sulfasalazine

Sulfasalazine frequently produces adverse effects; however, they are usually not severe. Patients may experience anorexia, nausea, vomiting, dyspepsia, diarrhea, fatigue, headaches, and skin eruptions. In the studies noted above, the majority of the patients were able to tolerate the medication [74, 75]. Gupta et al. noted the adverse effects that occurred in their open-label study patients were usually mild and temporary. Eight (25%) patients did not complete the study due to noncompliance (2), a likely drug-induced macular eruption (4), nausea and fatigue (1), and elevated liver function tests (1) [75]. Gastrointestinal symptoms, specifically nausea and vomiting, appear to be the most common side effect. Patients who cannot tolerate these effects may be given enteric-coated tablets [9]. In the studies cited above, 17–19% of the subjects developed a reversible cutaneous drug reaction [74, 75]. Generally, this reaction appears as a pruritic diffuse erythematous maculopapular eruption; it may be photodistributed [9, 75]. Patients may experience photosensitivity [74]; therefore, caution should be used when combining sulfasalazine with other photosensitizing agents or phototherapy. Potentially fatal hepatotoxicity including elevated liver function tests, jaundice, cirrhosis and necrosis has been reported [78]. Hematological effects including hemolytic anemia, aplastic anemia leukopenia, neutropenia, thrombocytopenia, and agranulocytosis may occur [9, 78]. The only statistically significant lab abnormality noted in the double-blind study by Gupta et al. was a decreased hemoglobin which was not clinically significant as per the authors [74]. Sulfasalazine is pregnancy category B.

Combination, rotational, and sequential therapy

A systemic agent may be used in combinations with other systemic therapies, topical therapies or phototherapy. Concurrent use may result in a more rapid response while using lower doses of each medication thereby reducing the incidence of side effects. Common combinations include retinoids plus psoralen ultraviolet-A (PUVA) or ultraviolet-B therapy (UV-B) therapy, methotrexate plus UV-B, PUVA plus UV-B, or methotrexate plus cyclosporine [10]. For thick-plaque psoriasis, acitretin with either PUVA or UV-B has shown excellent results. These combinations may be especially useful in areas that are generally poorly responsive to treatment, such as the scalp, palms, and soles [11, 79]. Methotrexate may be added to acitretin monotherapy to achieve a rapid clearance and discontinued once the patient is cleared [11]. Rotational therapy involves rotating single agents to minimize total cumulative doses [80]. Sequential therapy is the use of different therapies, topical or systemic, in sequence. It takes advantage of the fact that psoriatic lesions respond rapidly to some medications while other medications serve as better maintenance regimens. This approach is comprised of three phases: (1) the clearing phase, (2) the transitional phase, and (3) the maintenance phase. There is an overlap of the rapidly acting drug and the maintenance drug during the second phase. This phase may be the most difficult to manage because exacerbations may occur as the rapidly acting medication is tapered and the maintenance therapy is adjusted [81].

References

1 Napoli JL, Boerman MH, Chai X, Zhai Y, Fiorella PD (1995) Enzymes and binding proteins affecting retinoic acid concentrations. *J Steroid Biochem Mol Biol* 53: 497–502
2 Napoli JL (1996) Retinoic acid biosynthesis and metabolism. *FASEB J* 10: 993–1001
3 Saurat JH (1999) Retinoids and psoriasis: novel issues in retinoid pharmacology and implications for psoriasis treatment. *J Am Acad Dermatol* 41: S2–6
4 Torma H, Rollman O, Vahlquist A (1998) Interferon-γ increases retinoic acid and 3,4-didehydroretinoic acid concentrations in cultured keratinocytes: a clue to the abnormal vitamin A metabolism in psoriatic skin. *J Invest Dermatol* 110: 551
5 Geiger JM, Saurat JH (1993) Acitretin and etretinate. How and when they should be used. *Dermatol Clin* 11: 117–129
6 Ling MR (1999) Acitretin: optimal dosing strategies. *J Am Acad Dermatol* 41: S13–17
7 Soriatane package insert (2004) Palo Alto, CA: Connectics Corporation
8 Geiger JM, Czarnetzki BM (1988) Acitretin (Ro 10-1670, etretin): overall evaluation of clinical studies. *Dermatologica* 176: 182–190
9 Camisa C (2004) *Handbook of psoriasis*. Publishing Ltd, Malden, MA
10 Lebwohl M, Ali S (2001) Treatment of psoriasis. Part 2. Systemic therapies. *J Am Acad Dermatol* 45: 649–661
11 Roenigk HH (1999) Acitretin combination therapy. *J Am Acad Dermatol* 41: S18–21
12 Katz HI, Waalen J, Leach EE (1999) Acitretin in psoriasis: an overview of adverse effects. *J Am Acad Dermatol* 41: S7–S12
13 McNamara PJ, Jewell RC, Jensen BK, Brindley CJ (1988) Food increases the bioavailability of acitretin. *J Clin Pharmacol* 28: 1051–1055

14 Nguyen EQH (2001) Systemic retinoids. In: CL Kulp-Shorten, SE Wolverton (eds): *Comprehensive dermatologic drug therapy*. WB Saunders Company, Philadelphia (PA), 269–310
15 McClure SL, Valentine J, Gordon KB (2002) Comparative tolerability of systemic treatments for plaque-type psoriasis. *Drug Saf* 25: 913–927
16 Roche Laboratories, data on file
17 Gollnick HP (1996) Oral retinoids: efficacy and toxicity in psoriasis. *Br J Dermatol* 135 Suppl 49: 6–17
18 Wilson DJ, Kay V, Charig M, Hughes DG, Creasy TS (1988) Skeletal hyperostosis and extraosseous calcification in patients receiving long-term etretinate (Tigason). *Br J Dermatol* 119: 597–607
19 Yarbro JW (1969) Hydroxyurea in the treatment of refractory psoriasis. *Lancet* 2: 846–847
20 Leavell UW, Yarbro JW (1970) Hydroxyurea. A new treatment for psoriasis. *Arch Dermatol* 102: 144–150
21 Yamauchi PS, Rizk D, Kormeili T, Patnail R, Lowe NJ (2003) Current systemic therapies for psoriasis: where are we now? *J Am Acad Dermatol* 49: S66–77
22 Vogler WR, Bain JA, Huguley CM (1966) *In vivo* effect of hydroxyurea on orotic acid synthesis. *Cancer Res* 26: 1827–1831
23 Klem EB (1978) Effects of antipsoriasis drugs and metabolic inhibitors on the growth of epidermal cells in culture. *J Invest Dermatol* 70: 27–32
24 Boyd AS, Neldner KH (1991) Hydroxyurea therapy. *J Am Acad Dermatol* 25: 518–524
25 Burns DA, Sarkany I, Gaylarde P (1980) Effects of hydroxyurea therapy on normal skin: a case report. *Clin Exp Dermatol* 5: 447–449
26 Kennedy BJ, Smith LR, Goltx RW (1975) Skin changes secondary to hydroxyurea therapy. *Arch Dermatol* 111: 183–187
27 Stein KM, Shelley WB, Weinberg RA (1971) Hydroxyurea in the treatment of pustular psoriasis. *Br J Dermatol* 85: 81–85
28 Wahba A, Cohen H, Bar-Eli M, Callily R (1979) Neutrophil chemotaxis in psoriasis. *Acta Derm Venereol* 59: 441–445
29 Moschella SL, Greenwald MA (1973) Psoriasis with hydroxyurea. An 18-month study of 60 patients. *Arch Dermatol* 107: 363–368
30 Layton AM, Sheehan-Dare RA, Goodfield MJ, Cotterill JA (1989) Hydroxyurea in the management of therapy resistant psoriasis. *Br J Dermatol* 121: 647–653
31 Kumar B, Saraswat A, Kaur I (2001) Rediscovering hydroxyurea: its role in recalcitrant psoriasis. *Int J Dermatol* 40: 530–534
32 Hydrea package insert (2001) Princeton, NJ: Bristol-Myers Squibb Company
33 Kumar B, Saraswat A, Kaur I (2002) Mucocutaneous adverse effects of hydroxyurea: a prospective study of 30 psoriasis patients. *Clin Exp Dermatol* 27: 8–13
34 Thurman WG, Bloedow C, Howe CD, Levin WC, Davis P, Lane M, Sullivan MP, Griffith KM (1963) A phase I study of hydroxyurea. *Cancer Chemother Rep* 29: 103–107
35 Folan DW (1977) Severe reaction to hydroxyurea. *Cutis* 20: 95
36 Heddle R, Calvert AF (1980) Hydroxyurea induced hepatitis. *Med J Aust* 1: 121
37 Baker H (1982) Antimitotic drugs in psoriasis. In: EM Farber, AJ Cox (eds): *Psoriasis: Proceedings of the Third International Symposium*. Grune and Stratton, New York, 119–126
38 Samuels ML, Howe CD (1964) Renal abnormalities induced by hydroxyurea (NSC-32065) *Cancer Chemother Rep* 40: 9–13
39 Snow JL, Gibson LE (1995) The role of genetic variation in thiopurine methyltransferase activity and the efficacy and/or side effects of azathioprine therapy in dermatologic patients. *Arch Dermatol* 131: 193–197
40 Kazlow Stern D, Tripp JM, Ho VC, Lebwohl M (2005) The use of systemic immune moderators in dermatology: an update. *Dermatol Clin* 23: 259–300
41 Sanderson J, Ansari A, Marinaki T, Duley J (2004) Thiopurine methyltransferase: should it be measured before commencing thiopurine drug therapy? *Ann Clin Biochem* 41: 294–302
42 Patel AA, Swerlick RA, McCall CO (2006) Azathioprine in dermatology: the past, the present, and the future. *J Am Acad Dermatol* 55: 369–389
43 35. Holme SA, Duley JA, Sanderson J, Routledge PA, Anstey AV (2002) Erythrocyte thiopurine methyl transferase assessment prior to azathioprine use in the UK. *QJM* 95: 439–444
44 Weinshilboum RM, Sladek SL (1980) Mercaptopurine pharmacogenetics: monogenic inheritance of erythrocyte thiopurine methyltransferase activity. *Am J Hum Genet* 32: 651–662

45 du Vivier A, Munro DD, Verbov J (1974) Treatment of psoriasis with azathioprine. *Br Med J* 1: 49–51
46 Zackheim HS, Glogau RG, Fisher DA, Maibach HI (1994) 6-Thioguanine treatment of psoriasis: experience in 81 patients. *J Am Acad Dermatol* 30: 452–458
47 Mason C, Krueger GG (2001) Thioguanine for refractory psoriasis: a 4-year experience. *J Am Acad Dermatol* 44: 67–72
48 Anstey AV, Wakelin S, Reynolds NJ (2004) Guidelines for prescribing azathioprine in dermatology. *Br J Dermatol* 151: 1123–1132
49 Tabloid package insert (2004) Research Triangle Park, NC: GlaxoSmithKline
50 Silvis NG, Levine N (1999) Pulse dosing of thioguanine in recalcitrant psoriasis. *Arch Dermatol* 135: 433–437
51 Imuran package insert (2001) San Diego, CA: Prometheus Laboratories, Inc.
52 Kao NL, Rosenblate HJ (1993) 6-Thioguanine therapy for psoriasis causing toxic hepatic venoocclusive disease. *J Am Acad Dermatol* 28: 1017–1018
53 de Boer NK, Jarbandhan SV, de Graaf P, Mulder CJ, van Elburg RM, van Bodegraven AA (2006) Azathioprine use during pregnancy: unexpected intrauterine exposure to metabolites. *Am J Gastroenterol* 101: 1390–1392
54 de Boer NK, van Elburg RM, Wilhelm AJ, Remmink AJ, van Vugt JM, Mulder CJ, van Bodegraven AA (2005) 6-Thioguanine for Crohn's disease during pregnancy: thiopurine metabolite measurements in both mother and child. *Scand J Gastroenterol* 40: 1374–1377
55 Norgard B, Pedersen L, Jacobsen J, Rasmussen SN, Sorensen HT (2004) The risk of congenital abnormalities in children fathered by men treated with azathioprine or mercaptopurine before conception. *Aliment Pharmacol Ther* 19: 679–685
56 Rajapakse RO, Korelitz BI, Zlatanic J, Baiocco PJ, Gleim GW (2000) Outcome of pregnancies when fathers are treated with 6-mercaptopurine for inflammatory bowel disease. *Am J Gastroenterol* 95: 684–688
57 Allison AC, Eugui EM (1996) Purine metabolism and immunosuppressive effects if mycophenolate mofetil (MMF). *Clin Transplant* 10: 77–84
58 Geilen CC, Arnold M, Orfanos CE (2001) Mycophenolic mofetil as a systemic antipsoriatic agent: positive experience in 11 patients. *Br J Dermatol* 144: 583–586
59 Kitchin JE, Pomeranz MK, Pak G, Washenik K, Shupack JL (1997) Rediscovering mycophenolic acid: a review of its mechanism, side effects, and potential uses. *J Am Acad Dermatol* 37: 445–449
60 Jones EL, Epinette WW, Hackney VC, Menendez L, Frost P (1975) Treatment of psoriasis with oral mycophenolic acid. *J Invest Dermatol* 65: 537–542
61 Lynch WS, Roenigk HH (1977) Mycophenolic acid for psoriasis. *Arch Dermatol* 113: 1203–1208
62 Marinari R, Fleischmajer R, Schragger AH, Rosenthal AL (1977) Mycophenolic acid in the treatment of psoriasis: long-term administration. *Arch Dermatol* 113: 930–932
63 Gomez EC, Menendez L, Frost P (1979) Efficacy of mycophenolic acid for the treatment of psoriasis. *J Am Acad Dermatol* 1: 531–537
64 Epinette WW, Parker CM, Jones EL, Greist MC (1987) Mycophenolic acid for psoriasis. A review of pharmacology, long-term efficacy, and safety. *J Am Acad Dermatol* 17: 962–971
65 Haufs MG, Beissert S, Grabbe S, Schutte B, Luger TA (1998) Psoriasis vulgaris treated successfully with mycophenolate mofetil. *Br J Dermatol* 138: 179–181
66 Zhou Y, Rosenthal D, Dutz J, Ho V (2003) Mycophenolate mofetil (CellCept) for psoriasis: a two-center, prospective, open-label clinical trial. *J Cutan Med Surg* 7: 193–197
67 CellCept package insert (2005) Nutley, NJ: Roche Laboratories
68 Myfortic package insert (2004) East Hanover, NJ: Novartis Pharmaceuticals Corporation
69 Mathew TH (1998) A blinded, long-term, randomized multicenter study of mycophenolate mofetil in cadaveric renal transplantation: results at three years. Tricontinental Mycophenolate Mofetil Renal Transplantation Study Group. *Transplantation* 65: 1450–1454
70 Platz KP, Sollinger HW, Hullett DA, Eckhoff DE, Eugui EM, Allison AC (1991) RS-61443 – a new, potent immunosuppressive agent. *Transplantation* 51: 27–31
71 Ensley RD, Bristow MR, Olsen SL, Taylor DO, Hammond DH, O'Connell JB, Dunn D, Osburn L, Jones KW, Kauffman RS et al. (1993) The use of mycophenolate mofetil (RS-61443) in human heart transplant recipients. *Transplantation* 56: 75–82
72 Goldblum R (1993) Therapy of rheumatoid arthritis with mycophenolate mofetil. *Clin Exper Rheum* 11: S117–119
73 Cohen HD, Das KM (2006) The metabolism of mesalamine and its possible use in colonic diver-

ticulitis as an anti-inflammatory agent. *J Clin Gastroenterol* 40: S150–154
74 Gupta AK, Ellis CN, Siegel MT, Duell EA, Griffiths CE, Hamilton TA, Nickoloff BJ, Voorhees JJ (1990) Sulfasalazine improves psoriasis. A double-blind analysis. *Arch Dermatol* 126: 487–493
75 Gupta AK, Ellis CN, Siegel MT, Voorhees JJ (1989) Sulfasalazine: a potential psoriasis therapy? *J Am Acad Dermatol* 20: 797–800
76 Schoch EP, McCuistion CH (1955) The effect of salicylazosulfapyridine (azulfidine) on pustular acne vulgaris and certain other dermatoses. *J Invest Dermatol* 25: 123–126
77 Lorincz AL, Pearson RW (1962) Sulfapyridine and sulfone type drugs in dermatology. *Arch Dermatol* 85: 2–16
78 Azulfidine package insert (2002) Kalamazoo, MI: Pharmacia Corporation
79 Lebwohl M (1999) Acitretin in combination with UVB or PUVA. *J Am Acad Dermatol* 41: S22–24
80 Weinstein GD, White GM (1993) An approach to the treatment of moderate to severe psoriasis with rotational therapy. *J Am Acad Dermatol* 28: 454–459
81 Koo J (1999) Systemic sequential therapy of psoriasis: a new paradigm for improved therapeutic results. *J Am Acad Dermatol* 41: S25–28

Biologic therapy for psoriasis: an overview of infliximab, etanercept, adalimumab, efalizumab, and alefacept

Jeffrey M. Weinberg

Department of Dermatology, St. Luke's-Roosevelt Hospital Center and Beth Israel Medical Center, New York, NY, USA

Introduction

The implication of an immunologic phenomena in the pathogenesis of psoriasis has led to research for new treatment options over the past few years [1]. The result has been the birth of biologic therapies, those drugs targeting the activity of T lymphocytes and cytokines responsible for the inflammatory nature of this disease. Singri et al. [2] defined four strategies that clarify the mechanism of action for the various biologic agents: (1) reduction of pathogenic T cells, (2) inhibition of T cell activation, (3) immune deviation ('deviation' of a T_H1 immune response toward a greater T_H2-type response through the involvement of these T_H2-type cytokines), and (4) blocking the activity of inflammatory cytokines [2]. We have previously reviewed the utility of biologic agents for psoriasis [3]. In this article, we present an update on the progress of the tumor necrosis factor inhibitors infliximab, etanercept, and adalimumab (all strategy 4) as well as the T cell-targeted therapies efalizumab (strategy 2) and alefacept (strategy 1) (Tab. 1). Clinical data for these agents, including the most recent Phase II and/or III study results will be discussed, as well as the most recent safety data (Tab. 2).

Efficacy

Infliximab (Remicade®)

Infliximab is a chimeric (mouse-human) IgG1 monoclonal antibody that binds to tumor necrosis factor α (TNF-α). It also inhibits production of other pro-inflammatory cytokines, reducing cell infiltration and eventually keratinocyte proliferation. The drug is currently approved for Crohn's disease (CD), psoriasis, psoriatic arthritis, and rheumatoid arthritis (RA), as an intravenous infusion.

Recently, Gottlieb et al. [4] assessed the efficacy and safety of infliximab induction therapy for patients with severe plaque psoriasis. In this multicenter,

Table 1 Summary of biologic agents for psoriasis

Agent	Mechanism of action	Administration	Status
Infliximab	TNF-α inhibitor-chimeric antibody	IV infusion (>120 min)	FDA approved for psoriasis, oriatic arthritis
Etanercept	TNF-α inhibitor-TNF receptor	SC twice weekly	FDA approved for psoriasis, psoriatic arthritis
Adalimumab	TNF-α inhibitor-human antibody	SC once weekly/every other week	Submitted to FDA for psoriasis, FDA approved for psoriatic arthritis
Efalizumab	Inhibits T cell activation, migration	SC once weekly	FDA approved for psoriasis
Alefacept	Reduces memory-effector T cells	IM once weekly	FDA approved for psoriasis

Table 2 Efficacy of biologic agents

Agent	Dose (duration)	PASI 50	PASI 75	PASI 90
Infliximab				
Phase III	5 mg/kg (0,2,6 wk, then every 8 wks)	10 weeks: 91%	10 weeks: 80%	10 weeks: 57%
		24 weeks: 90%	24 weeks: 82%	24 weeks: 58%
		50 weeks: 69%	50 weeks: 61%	50 weeks: 45%
Etanercept				
Phase III	25 mg SC 2X/wk (24 wk)	12 weeks: 58%	12 weeks: 34%	12 weeks: 12%
		24 weeks: 70%	24 weeks: 44%	24 weeks: 20%
	50 mg SC 2X/wk (24 wk)	12 weeks: 74%	12 weeks: 49%	12 weeks: 22%
		24 weeks: 77%	24 weeks: 59%	24 weeks: 30%
Adalimumab				
Phase II	80 mg wk 0, 1 then 40 mg qwk (12 wk)	12 weeks: 88%	12 weeks: 80%	12 weeks: 48%
		24 weeks: NA	24 weeks: 77%	24 weeks: 66%
		60 weeks: 75%	60 weeks: 73%	60 weeks: 55%
	80 mg wk 0, 1 then 40 mg every other wk (12 wk)	12 weeks: 76%	12 weeks: 53%	12 weeks: 24%
		24 weeks: NA	24 weeks: 69%	24 weeks: 44%
		60 weeks: 76%	60 weeks: 67%	60 weeks: 36%
Efalizumab				N/A
Phase III	1 mg/kg/wk (12wk)	12 weeks: 57.0%	12 weeks: 27.9%	
	2 mg/kg/wk (12 wk)	12 weeks: 54.5%	12 weeks: 27.6%	
Phase III	1 mg/kg/wk (24 wk)	12 weeks: 58.5%	12 weeks: 26.6%	
		24 weeks: 66.6%	24 weeks: 43.8%	
Alefacept IM	15 mg IM (12 wk)	14 weeks: 42%	14 weeks: 21%	N/A
Phase III	15 mg IM (12 wk)	Any Time: 57%	Any Time: 33%	

double-blind, placebo-controlled trial, 249 patients with severe plaque psoriasis were randomly assigned to receive intravenous infusions of either 3 or 5 mg/kg of infliximab or placebo given at weeks 0, 2, and 6. The primary endpoint was the proportion of patients who achieved at least 75% improvement in Psoriasis Area and Severity Index (PASI) score from baseline at week 10. At week 26, patients whose Physician Global Assessment indicated moderate or severe disease were eligible for a single intravenous infusion of their assigned treatment to assess the safety of re-treatment after a 20-week, treatment-free interval [2].

At week 10, 72% of patients treated with infliximab (3 mg/kg) and 88% of patients treated with infliximab (5 mg/kg) achieved a 75% or greater improvement from baseline in PASI score compared with 6% of patients treated with placebo ($P < .001$). Improvement was observed in both infliximab groups as early as 2 weeks. Overall, 63%, 78%, and 79% of patients in the placebo, 3-, and 5-mg/kg groups, respectively, reported one or more adverse events. The authors concluded that infliximab treatment resulted in a rapid and significant improvement in the signs and symptoms of psoriasis. In addition, infliximab was generally well tolerated [2].

Reich et al. [5] assessed the efficacy and safety of continuous treatment with infliximab in a Phase III, multicenter, double-blind trial. In this study, 378 patients with moderate-to-severe plaque psoriasis were allocated in a 4:1 ratio to receive infusions of either infliximab 5 mg/kg or placebo at weeks 0, 2, and 6, then every 8 weeks to week 46. At week 24, placebo-treated patients crossed over to infliximab treatment. Skin and nail signs of psoriasis were assessed using PASI index and nail psoriasis severity index (NAPSI), respectively. The primary endpoint, analyzed on an intention-to-treat-basis, was the proportion of patients achieving at least a 75% improvement in PASI from baseline to week 10. At week 10, 80% (242/301) of patients treated with infliximab achieved at least a 75% improvement from their baseline PASI (PASI 75) and 57% (172/301) achieved at least a 90% improvement (PASI 90), compared with 3% and 1% in the placebo group, respectively ($p < 0.0001$). At week 24, PASI 75 (82% for infliximab *versus* 4% for placebo) and PASI 90 (58% *versus* 1%) were maintained ($p < 0.0001$). At week 50, 61% achieved PASI 75 and 45% achieved PASI 90 in the infliximab group. Infliximab was generally well tolerated in most patients. Infliximab is effective in both an induction and maintenance regimen for the treatment of moderate-to-severe psoriasis, with a high percentage of patients achieving sustained PASI 75 and PASI 90 improvement through 1 year [5].

Etanercept (Enbrel®)

Etanercept is a 100% human TNF-receptor, made from the fusion of two naturally occurring TNF-receptors. It binds to TNF with greater affinity than natural receptors, which are monomeric. The binding of etanercept to TNF renders the bound TNF biologically inactive, resulting in reduction in inflammatory activity. Etanercept is administered subcutaneously by patients at home. The drug is approved for rheumatoid arthritis (RA), juvenile rheumatoid arthritis, ankylosing sponylitis, psoriasis, and psoriatic arthritis. Etanercept is also indicated for inhibiting the progression of structural damage and improving physical function in patients with RA and psoriatic arthritis, and improving physical function in patients with RA. The approved dose in psoriasis is 50 mg subcutaneously twice weekly for 3 months, followed by 25 mg twice weekly subcutaneously.

The results of a Phase III study evaluating the efficacy and tolerability of etanercept in psoriasis were recently reported [6]. Etanercept was evaluated at doses of 25 mg and 50 mg subcutaneously twice weekly. At the 25 mg dose, the percentage of patients achieving PASI 75 was 34% at 12 weeks and 49% at 24 weeks. At the 50 mg dose, the percentage of patients achieving PASI 75 was 49% at 12 weeks and 59% at 24 weeks. Therapy with etanercept was generally well tolerated [6].

Papp et al. [7] performed a Phase III study to further examine the efficacy and safety of etanercept, and to assess maintenance of treatment effect after dose reduction of etanercept. This was a multicenter 24-week study conducted in the US, Canada and Western Europe. During the first 12 weeks of the study, patients were randomly assigned to receive by subcutaneous injection etanercept twice weekly (BIW) at a dose of 50 mg or 25 mg, or placebo BIW in a double-blind fashion. During the second 12 weeks, all patients received etanercept 25 mg BIW. The primary endpoint was a 75% or greater improvement from baseline PASI at 12 weeks. 583 subjects were randomized and received at least one dose of study drug. At week 12, a PASI 75 was achieved by 49% of patients in the etanercept 50 mg BIW group, 34% in the 25 mg BIW group, and 3% in the placebo group ($P < 0.0001$ for each etanercept group compared with placebo). At week 24 (after 12 weeks of open-label 25 mg etanercept BIW), a PASI 75 was achieved by 54% of patients whose dose was reduced from 50 mg BIW to 25 mg BIW, by 45% of patients in the continuous 25 mg BIW group, and by 28% in the group that received placebo followed by etanercept 25 mg BIW. Etanercept was well tolerated throughout the study. The authors concluded that etanercept provided clinically meaningful benefit to patients with chronic plaque psoriasis, with no apparent decrease in efficacy after dose reduction [7].

Magliocco and Gottlieb [8] reported three cases of use of etanercept in patients with hepatitis C. Psoriasis and psoriatic arthritis are exacerbated by interferon-α and other treatments for hepatitis C virus infection. Immunosuppressants and hepatotoxic drugs are relatively contraindicated in hepatitis C [8]. Data in the literature suggest that etanercept is a safe option in the treatment of patients with rheumatoid arthritis and concurrent hepatitis C. The authors presented three cases in which they successfully used etanercept to treat psoriatic arthritis/psoriasis in patients with hepatitis C without worsening their hepatitis or interfering with their hepatitis treatment. With close monitoring of viral load and hepatic enzymes, the authors concluded that etanercept may be a safe option for treating psoriatic arthritis/psoriasis in patients who also have hepatitis C [8].

Adalimumab (Humira®)

Adalimumab is a human IgG1 monoclonal tumor necrosis factor alpha (TNF-α) antibody [9]. The binding of adalimumab to TNF-α results in its inactivation, thus reducing inflammatory activity. Adalimumab is currently approved for the treatment of psoriatic arthritis, and has completed Phase III clinical trials for its potential use in the treatment of psoriasis. It can be administered like etanercept, via subcutaneous injection.

Gordon et al. [10] recently reported preliminary efficacy and safety data from a 12-week, double-blind, placebo-controlled Phase II trial of adalimumab in psoriasis. The researchers enrolled 148 adults with a diagnosis of moderate to severe chronic plaque psoriasis for at least 1 year and an affected body area (BSA) of 5% or greater. The subjects were randomized to two active treatment groups and one placebo group. All subjects were naive to TNF-antagonist treatment. In the year prior to entry, about 40% of subjects had used methotrexate, cyclosporine, or an oral retinoid; 16% had used a biologic therapy approved for psoriasis; and 26% had undergone phototherapy.

One group of subjects received 80 mg adalimumab at week 0, followed by 40 mg every other week from week 1 onward. The second active group received 80 mg at weeks 0 and 1, then 40 mg weekly beginning at week 2. Placebo was administered weekly to the third group. 95% of the subjects completed the study. The primary endpoint was the percentage of subjects achieving at least a 75% reduction in the psoriasis area and severity index (PASI) at week 12. Adalimumab 40 mg every other week achieved a mean PASI greater than or equal to 75 at a 53% rate compared with a 4% rate for placebo, and 40 mg weekly achieved a mean PASI greater than or equal to 75 at an 80% rate [10].

The results for this trial at 60 weeks were also recently reported [11]. Upon completion of 12 weeks of therapy, patients in the treatment group were eligible to continue their assigned blinded dose, adalimumab 40 mg either weekly or every other week, while the placebo group was switched to an 80 mg loading dose of adalimumab at week 12 and then 40 mg every other week, starting at week 13.

In the study, 67% of patients on adalimumab 40 mg every other week achieved at least a 75% improvement in PASI after 60 weeks. Furthermore, after 60 weeks more than one-third (36%) of patients in the adalimumab 40 mg every other week group achieved PASI 90. Additionally, almost two-thirds (63%) of patients were determined to be ‘clear’ or ‘almost clear’ of their psoriasis as measured by the Physician’s Global Assessment, another measurement tool used by physicians to assess severity of disease.

Patients also recorded significant improvement in quality of life measures after 60 weeks of treatment with the adalimumab 40 mg every other week group with 34.3% of patients reporting their quality of life was 'not at all' affected by their psoriasis, as measured by the Dermatology Life Quality Index (DLQI) [11].

Safety

The TNF-inhibitors share a number of common safety issues and concerns. These include infection, risk of lymphoma, demyelinating disease, heart failure, and drug-induced lupus.

Infection

Infection is an issue of major concern, and there have been multiple reports of reactivation of latent tuberculosis with infliximab (TB) [12–14]. The available *in vitro* and epidemiological evidence for the TNF inhibitors infliximab and etanercept, shows that the risk of development of active tuberculosis is higher with infliximab [15]. In controlled trials, however, an increased risk of serious infection in infliximab-treated patients has not been observed [12].

Hamilton [16] recently reviewed the infectious complications of biologic therapy. His review described the most important pathogen-specific infections and their relative frequency. Tuberculosis has continued to be the most common pathogen reported in association with infliximab, and less so with etanercept and adalimumab. Determining treated population case rates depends on having an accurate denominator and reflects the local population's latent infection rate. The same is true for histoplasmosis. Other pathogens requiring intact cellular immunity for control of latent infection have also been reported. Specific recommendations for preventive therapy are being made, but prospective clinical trials are needed to assess the risk-benefit of any particular approach. He concluded that microorganisms responsible for the infectious complications associated with anticytokine therapy are generally intracellular pathogens or pathogens that commonly exist in a chronic, latent state and are normally held in check by cell-mediated immunity. Diagnosis requires a high index of suspicion and prompt acquisition of appropriate tissue for microscopic examination and microbiologic culture [16]. A PPD is required prior to the use of adalimumab and infliximab, and many clinicians utilize a PPD before the initiation of etanercept.

Lymphoma

One of the major concerns with the use of TNF inhibitors is the potential risk for development of lymphomas. Brown et al. [17] investigated the occurrence of lymphoproliferative disorders in patients treated with these agents. They reviewed relevant data in the MedWatch post-market adverse event surveillance system run by the US Food and Drug Administration (FDA) and identified 26 cases of lymphoproliferative disorders following treatment with etanercept (18 cases) or infliximab (8 cases). The majority of cases (81%) were non-Hodgkin's lymphomas. The interval between initiation of therapy with etanercept or infliximab and the development of lymphoma was very short (median 8 weeks). The authors concluded that, although data from a case series such theirs cannot establish a clear causal relationship between exposure to these medications and the risk of lymphoproliferative disease, the known predisposition of patients with diseases such as RA and CD to lymphoma, the known excess of lymphoma in other immunosuppressed populations, and the known immunosuppressive effects of the anti-TNF drugs, provide a biologic basis for concern and justification for the initiation of additional epidemiologic studies to formally evaluate this possible association [17].

The risk of lymphoma is increased in patients with rheumatoid arthritis (RA), and spontaneous reporting suggests that methotrexate (MTX) and anti-tumor necrosis factor (anti-TNF) therapy might be associated independently with an increased risk of lymphoma [18]. Wolfe and Michaud [18] conducted a study to determine the rate of and standardized incidence ratio (SIR) for lymphoma in patients with RA and in RA patient subsets by treatment group. Additionally, they sought to determine predictors of lymphoma in RA. They prospectively studied 18'572 patients with RA who were enrolled in the National Data Bank for Rheumatic Diseases (NDB). Patients were surveyed biannually, and potential lymphoma cases received detailed follow up. The SEER (Survey, Epidemiology, and End Results) cancer data resource was used to derive the expected number of cases of lymphoma in a cohort that was comparable in age and sex with the RA cohort [18].

The overall SIR for lymphoma was 1.9 (95% confidence interval [95% CI] 1.3–2.7). The SIR for biologic use was 2.9 (95% CI 1.7–4.9) and for the use of infliximab (with or without etanercept) was 2.6 (95% CI 1.4–4.5). For etanercept, with or without infliximab, the SIR was 3.8 (95% CI 1.9–7.5). The SIR for MTX was 1.7 (95% CI 0.9–3.2), and was 1.0 (95% CI 0.4–2.5) for those not receiving MTX or biologics. Lymphoma was associated with increasing age, male sex, and education. The authors concluded that lymphomas are increased in RA. Although the SIR is greatest for anti-TNF therapies, differences between therapies are slight, and confidence intervals for treatment groups overlap. The increased lymphoma rates observed with anti-TNF therapy may reflect channeling bias, whereby patients with the highest risk of lymphoma preferentially receive anti-TNF therapy. Current data are insufficient to establish a causal relationship between RA treatments and the development of lymphoma [18].

Adams et al. [19] described two cases of cutaneous and systemic T cell lymphoma that progressed rapidly in the setting of TNF-α blockade, one with etanercept and one with infliximab. Both cases were characterized by rapid onset, a fulminant clinical course with extensive cutaneous and systemic involvement, and death within months of diagnosis.

A warning was recently added to infliximab's package insert [20]. Data from studies showed a six-fold lymphoma increase among rheumatoid arthritis and Crohn's disease patients taking the drug. The studies showed a three-fold increase among arthritis patients alone. The studies suggest that the combined population of rheumatoid arthritis and Crohn's disease patients taking infliximab will have 12 cases of lymphoma for every 10'000 patients taking the drug for 1 year. Among arthritis patients alone, there would be seven lymphoma cases for every 10'000 patients taking infliximab for 1 year [20].

The incidence of lymphomas seen in patients receiving adalimumab is similar to that of the general RA population. Among 2'468 rheumatoid arthritis patients treated in clinical trials with the drug for a median of 24 months, 10 patients with lymphoma were seen. The Standardized Incidence Ratio (SIR) (ratio of observed rate to age-adjusted expected frequency in the general population) for lymphomas was 5.4 (95% CI, 2.6, 10.0) [21].

Demyelinating disease

There have been infrequent reports of CNS demyelinating disorders during treatment with anti-TNF agents. Several of these cases have been temporally related to anti-TNF therapy and have resolved when treatment was withdrawn [22]. Mohan et al. [22] reviewed the occurrence of neurologic events suggestive of demyelination during anti-TNF therapy for inflammatory arthritides. The Adverse Events Reporting System of the FDA was queried following a report of a patient with refractory rheumatoid arthritis who developed confusion and difficulty with walking after receiving etanercept for 4 months. 19 patients with similar neurologic events were identified from the FDA database, 17 following etanercept administration and two following infliximab administration for inflammatory arthritis. All neurologic events were temporally related to anti-TNF therapy, with partial or complete resolution on discontinuation. One patient exhibited a positive rechallenge phenomenon. The authors concluded that further surveillance and studies are required to better define risk factors for and frequency of adverse events and their relationship to anti-TNF therapies. Until more long-term safety data are available, consideration should be given to avoiding anti-TNF therapy in patients with preexisting multiple sclerosis and to discontinuing anti-TNF therapy immediately when new neurologic signs and symptoms occur, pending an appropriate evaluation.

Given this data, etanercept, infliximab, or adalimumab should be avoided in patients with a personal history of any CNS demyelinating disorder and used with caution in patients with a family history of these disorders.

Heart failure

There have been rare reports of heart failure in patients receiving anti-TNF therapy, but the relationship to therapy is unclear because the background rate of heart failure may be elevated in the patient populations receiving these drugs [23]. Kwon et al. [23] utilizing the FDA's MedWatch program, documented 47 patients, who developed new or worsening heart failure during TNF antagonist therapy. After TNF antagonist therapy, 38 patients (26 etanercept, 12 infliximab) developed new-onset heart failure and nine patients (3 etanercept, 6 infliximab) experienced heart failure exacerbation. Of the 38 patients with new-onset heart failure, 19 (50%) (12 etanercept, 7 infliximab) had no identifiable risk factors. The authors concluded that, in a fraction of patients, TNF antagonists might induce new-onset heart failure or exacerbate existing disease. However, they noted that these spontaneous reports alone are not sufficient to make causal inferences [23].

Drug-induced lupus

Induction of antinuclear (ANA) and anti-DNA antibodies is observed in some patients treated with infliximab and etanercept [24]. Recently, the induction of true lupus erythematosus by TNF-inhibitors has been observed. Few cases without major organ involvement were reported to be associated with infliximab treatment that resolved after anti-TNF discontinuation [24–27] and only four cases have been described with the use of etanercept [28].

Drug-specific issues

Infliximab has been associated with a number of adverse events [12]. Infusion reactions, reported in 19% of patients in clinical trials, consist of fever or chills or more rarely chest pain, hypotension, hypertension, and dyspnea. Neutralizing antibodies are formed in a subset of patients, and are more likely to occur in patients who do not receive concurrent methotrexate. In addition, patients can develop a serum sickness reaction days after administration of the drug [12].

Etanercept has been used safely over the past few years. Injection site reactions are the main adverse events noted [12]. There have been infrequent observations of aplastic anemia and pancytopenia [12]. In etanercept clinical trials, <5% of patients developed antibodies, all of which were non-neutralizing.

Adalimumab has been associated with injection site reactions, with erythema, pain, swelling, itching, and hemorrhage, seen in 20% of patients [9]. The linkage of TNF-α inhibitors to the induction of autoantibodies is well known, with 12% of cases occurring following the use of adalimumab *versus* 7% in placebo. The incidence of less serious reactions like rash and pneumonia was significantly lower at 0.3% for both [9].

Efalizumab (Raptiva®)

Efalizumab is a humanized monoclonal antibody against the CD11a molecule. CD11a and CD18 comprise subunits of leukocyte function-associated antigen-1 (LFA-1), a T cell surface molecule important in T cell activation, T cell migration into skin, and cytotoxic T cell function. Binding of this drug to CD11a on T cells blocks the interaction between LFA-1 and ICAM-1, its partner molecule for adhesion. The blockade is reversible and does not deplete T cells.

Efficacy

Recently, a Phase III trial with subcutaneous (SC) efalizumab showed promising results in treatment of moderate to severe plaque psoriasis [29]. In this multicenter, randomized, placebo-controlled, double-blind study, 597 subjects with psoriasis were assigned to receive subcutaneous efalizumab (1 or 2 mg per kilogram of body weight per week) or placebo for 12 weeks. Depending on the response after 12 weeks, subjects received an additional 12 weeks of treatment with efalizumab or placebo. Study treatments were discontinued at week 24, and subjects were followed for an additional 12 weeks [29].

At week 12, there was an improvement of 75% or more in the PASI in 22% of the subjects who had received 1 mg of efalizumab per kilogram per week and 28% of those who had received 2 mg of efalizumab per kilogram per week, as compared with 5% of the subjects in the placebo group ($P < .001$ for both comparisons).

Efalizumab-treated subjects had greater improvement than those in the placebo group as early as week 4 ($P < .001$). Among the efalizumab-treated subjects who had an improvement of 75% or more at week 12, improvement was maintained through week 24 in 77% of those who continued to receive efalizumab, as compared with 20% of those who were switched to placebo ($P < .001$ for both comparisons).

After the discontinuation of efalizumab at week 24, an improvement of 50% or more in the PASI was maintained in approximately 30% of subjects during the 12 weeks of follow-up. Efalizumab was well tolerated, and adverse events were generally mild to moderate. The authors concluded that efalizumab therapy resulted in significant improvements in plaque psoriasis in subjects with moderate-to-severe disease. Extending treatment from 12 to 24 weeks resulted in both maintenance and improvement of responses [29].

Gordon et al. [30] assessed the efficacy and safety of efalizumab in patients with plaque psoriasis. In a Phase III randomized, double-blind, parallel-group, placebo-controlled trial involving 556 adult patients with stable, moderate to severe plaque psoriasis and conducted at 30 study centers in the US and Canada between January and July 2002, patients were randomly assigned in a 2:1 ratio to receive 12 weekly doses of subcutaneous efalizumab, 1 mg/kg (N = 369), or placebo equivalent (N = 187). The following were assessed: at least 75% improvement on the PASI; improvement on the overall Dermatology Life Quality Index (DLQI), Itching Visual Analog Scale (VAS), and Psoriasis Symptom Assessment (PSA) at week 12 *versus* baseline [30].

Efalizumab-treated patients experienced significantly greater improvement on all endpoints than placebo-treated patients. 27% of efalizumab-treated patients achieved PASI 75 *versus* 4% of the placebo group (P < .001). Efalizumab-treated patients exhibited significantly greater mean percentage improvement than placebo-treated patients on the overall DLQI (47% *versus* 14%; P < .001), Itching VAS (38% *versus* –0.2%; P < .001), and PSA frequency and severity subscales (48% *versus*.18% and 47% *versus*.17%, respectively; P < .001 for both) at the first assessment point. Efalizumab was safe and well tolerated with primarily mild to moderate adverse events [30].

Menter et al. [31] recently reported on the incidence and prevention of rebound of disease, following the discontinuation of efalizumab treatment in both a retrospective analysis of efalizumab clinical trials and in an open-label Phase IIIb transition study. Rebound is defined as worsening of psoriasis to 125% of the baseline PASI or the appearance of psoriasis variants such as erythrodermic or pustular psoriasis within 12 weeks of discontinuation of therapy. In the retrospective analysis, patient data from four efalizumab clinical trials were gathered to measure the incidence of rebound disease in patients with moderate to severe psoriasis during the 12-week treatment free follow-up period. The number of patients studied totaled 1'316 with all of them receiving a minimum of 12 weeks and up to 36 weeks of treatment. The patients who were placed in placebo groups (N = 479) (in the three studies which included placebo groups) were also separately analyzed for disease recurrence [31].

Results revealed that 14% (N = 188) of the patients that received efalizumab treatment suffered from rebound disease with the vast majority of recurrence being attributed to a PASI 125 (N = 182). The median length of time for occurrence of PASI 125 amounted to 36 days. On the other hand, 11% of the patients (N = 53) in the placebo group suffered rebound disease. Interestingly, of the 188 patients who experienced rebound, 72% of the patients were non-responders to efalizumab treatment, whereas only 18% of partial responders and 10% of responders to treatment experienced rebound. Despite the fact that these clinical trials had a 12-week washout period, certain patients were started on alternate therapeutic agents due to disease recurrence. Analysis was performed on the incidence of rebound disease in these patients. The results demonstrated that 91% of these patients (N = 578) that did have recurrence of disease did not rebound if they were treated with an alternative therapy [31].

In the multicenter, open-label Phase IIIb transition study 131 patients received a conditioning dose of 0.7 mg/kg of efalizumab followed by 11 weeks of 1 mg/kg of the drug. At the end of 12 weeks of treatment, patients were either placed in a group that received no treatment and were monitored for 12 weeks, or in a group that immediately received approved topical or systemic therapy and/or phototherapy for 12 weeks. Patients were placed in their respective groups based on how they responded by the end of week 12. The patients that received a _ 75% PASI (responders) score from baseline or a PGA score of 'excellent or clear' at the end of week 12 were placed in the group which did not receive alternative treatment. The patients with _ 50% PASI but less than 75% PASI (partial responders) and patients who did not achieve a 50% PASI (non responders) following therapy were placed in the group that received transition therapy with alternative agents. Of the 121 patients that were evaluated, 38% (N = 44) were classified as responders whereas 26% (N = 31) of patients were partial responders and 36% (N = 44) were considered non-responders. Of these patients, the responder group had no cases of rebound disease. On the other hand, 8% (N = 2) of the partial responder group and 22% (N = 8) of the non-responder group suffered from rebound disease. The median length of time for occurrence of rebound disease was 56 days for all the patients. These results reflected the findings of the retrospective analysis [31].

Toth and Papp [31] recently presented two case reports of patients with moderate to severe psoriasis who were effectively managed with alternate therapies following a rebound flare of disease subsequent to the discontinuation of efalizumab. Both patients had a long history of moderate to severe psoriasis and one had concomitant psoriatic arthritis. The two patients were enrolled in Phase III clinical trials and they received 1 mg/kg/wk of efalizumab for a period of 15 months in total. Subsequently, substantial improvement of psoriasis was observed in both cases. However, following the discontinuation of therapy, both patients experienced recurrence of disease. In the first case, disease reappearance occurred after 2 weeks, whereas in the second case reappearance occurred within 4 weeks of discontinuation. In response to the reemergence of disease, both patients were treated with 25 mg methotrexate. In addition, the patient in the first case was treated with betamethasone valerate 0.1% cream twice daily to affected areas on his body and hydrocortisone valerate cream twice daily for regions affected on his face. The patient in the second case received 5 mg of prednisone daily to specifically manage their concomitant flare up of disabling joint pain. In both cases the patient's flare of disease was attenuated and stabilized shortly thereafter with the first case stabilizing in 2 weeks and the second case stabilizing within 4 weeks. Following the initial stabilization, treatments with corticosteroids were tapered off. The patient in the first case was also able to be weaned off methotrexate 3 months after treatment initiation over a 4-week period. However, the patient in the second case was maintained on methotrexate with stable plaque psoriasis. In both cases, intervention with oral methotrexate and adjunct corticosteroid therapy successfully controlled the recurrence of psoriasis resulting from the cessation of efalizumab administration [32].

Safety

To date, very few serious adverse events have been reported in association with the T cell agents. The product labeling for efalizumab includes cautions about a potential increased risk of infection and malignancy, but an increase in the risk of either of these conditions has not been clearly demonstrated in either clinical trials or post-marketing surveillance. There have been no clinical signs of immunosuppression, and no hepatotoxicity or nephrotoxicity associated with the use of efalizumab [33]. In the Phase III trial, there was no evidence of T cell depletion or increased risk of end-organ toxicity, malignancy, or infection [29].

Efalizumab is very well tolerated, and the only significant safety concern is the risk of psoriasis worsening during or after discontinuation of therapy. In clinical trials, 14% of efalizumab-treated subjects who were abruptly withdrawn from treatment experienced rebound, which was defined previously [34]. Rebound following efalizumab discontinuation was much more likely to occur in patients who did not respond well to efalizumab, but it can occur in treatment responders as well. A further minor safety concern during efalizumab therapy is immune-mediated thrombocytopenia. During clinical trials for efalizumab, a small number of patients (8/2762; 0.3%) experienced reversible thrombocytopenia [34]. The causal relationship between efalizumab therapy and thrombocytopenia is unknown, but the product labeling recommends that platelet counts be obtained monthly for the first 3 months of efalizumab treatment, and every 3 months thereafter [34]. A recent warnings added to the package insert is the infrequent occurrence of immune-mediated hemolytic anemia. Infrequent severe arthritis events, including psoriatic arthritis, have also been reported [34].

Alefacept (Amevive®)

Psoriatic plaques are characterized by infiltration with $CD4^+$, $CD45RO^+$, $CD8^+$ and $CD45RO^+$ memory-effector T lymphocytes. The recombinant protein alefacept binds to CD2 on memory-effector T lymphocytes, inhibiting their activation and reducing the number of these cells. It is a fusion protein composed of leukocyte function-associated antigen type 3 (LFA-3) protein and human IgG1 Fc domains. The drug is administered by intramuscular injection.

Efficacy

An international multicenter trial randomized more than 500 patients to one of three arms: intramuscular (IM) alefacept 15 mg once a week for 12 weeks, IM alefacept 10 mg once a week for 12 weeks, or placebo [35]. 2 weeks after the last dose was given, 21% of patients treated with the 15-mg dose achieved at least a 75% reduction from baseline in their PASI score compared with 5% of patients receiving placebo ($P < .001$).

Krueger and Ellis [36] recently reported that alefacept therapy produces remission for patients with chronic plaque psoriasis. In the previously published randomized, placebo-controlled Phase II study of intravenous alefacept in 229 patients with chronic plaque psoriasis, clinical improvement was observed during dosing as well as in the post-dosing follow-up period [37]. Their objective was to assess the remission period following alefacept therapy in this population. In these patients, responses were sustained for a median of 10 months, and for up to 18 months. No patient reported disease rebound after cessation of alefacept [36].

Gribetz et al. [38] recently evaluated the safety and efficacy of an extended 16-week course of alefacept in patients with psoriasis. This single-center, Phase IV study enrolled 20 patients with psoriasis requiring either systemic therapy or phototherapy. The study included a 12-week open-label phase, followed by a 4-week double-blind phase and then an 8-week follow-up phase. The patients were randomly placed into two groups of 10 patients. In the open-label phase of the study, both groups received a 15 mg intramuscular (IM) injection of alefacept once weekly for 12 weeks. The following 4-week double-blind phase of the study consisted of Group 1 receiving weekly 15 mg IM injections of placebo and Group 2 receiving weekly 15 mg IM injections of alefacept for a total of four doses, respectively. The efficacy of the treatment was assessed using the change in PASI from baseline and Physician Global Assessment. The results revealed that there was a marked improvement in mean percentage change in PASI in both groups compared to baseline. The differences between the two groups, however, were not statistically significant. Between weeks 12 and 24, a total of six patients in each group achieved a PASI 50, whereas three patients in Group 2 achieved a PASI 75 compared to one patient in Group 1. Group 2 also had a higher mean percentage change (MPC) in PASI at week 12, and the MPC in PASI continued to increase through week 24 compared to the patients in Group 1. A statistically significant difference was found between the two groups at weeks 20 and 24 ($P < .05$; paired t-test). At 8 weeks post-treatment, only three patients had a PGA of 'clear' or 'almost clear', and these three patients were in Group 2. The results collected also showed that only one person in Group 1 had to have a dose suspended due to a low $CD4^+$ T cell count as apposed to two patients in Group 2. Of those two patients, one was withdrawn before week 12, and the other patient was withdrawn after week 12. In terms of safety and tolerability, no statistically significant difference in adverse events was found between the two groups from baseline to week 18 [38].

Safety

In terms of adverse events, patients treated with alefacept have a reduction in $CD45RO^+$ memory T cells, which correlates with improvement in psoriasis. To date, no clinically significant signs of immunosuppression or opportunistic infections have been observed, and no increase in malignancy has been observed [33]. In the US, weekly monitoring of T cells is recommended in patients treated with alefacept.

The product labeling for alefacept includes cautions about a potential increased risk of infection and malignancy, but an increase in the risk of either of these conditions has not been clearly demonstrated in either clinical trials or post-marketing surveillance [39]. There seem to be no serious safety concerns that are specific for alefacept. Alefacept does cause transient decreases in $CD4^+$ and $CD8^+$ cell counts, but there is no evidence that this significantly affects overall immune function. The product labeling for alefacept states that $CD4^+$ and $CD8^+$ cell counts must be monitored every 2 weeks during therapy, and that alefacept therapy should be withheld if counts are below 250 cells/μL (with weekly monitoring instituted) and suspended if counts stay below this level for a month or more [39].

Conclusion

Biologic therapy research continues to make great strides in the treatment of psoriasis. With continued progress at this rate, it is possible that one or more of these pharmacologic agents will become major therapeutic options for psoriasis. The data from this work is very encouraging, but we await further data from many of these medications, as well as those treatments which will follow.

These therapies offer successful therapy of psoriasis, with a lack of organ toxicity seen with traditional systemic therapies, such as methotrexate and cyclosporine. Limitations of the current data include the lack of direct head-to-head comparisons with traditional agents, and the absence of pharmacoeconomic evaluations of these agents, especially given the expected high costs of treatment. Long-term monitoring of these agents is necessary to determine the potential risk for increased infection and malignancy in patients treated with them.

Disclosure: Dr. Weinberg is a member of the Speaker's Bureau for Amgen, Abbott, and Genentech. There was no industry support for preparation and publication of this manuscript.

References

1 Tutrone WD, Kagen MH, Barbagallo J, Weinberg JM (2001) Biologic therapy for psoriasis: a brief history, II. *Cutis* 68: 367–372
2 Singri P, West DP, Gordon KB (2002) Biologic therapy for psoriasis: the new therapeutic frontier. *Arch Dermatol* 138: 657–663
3 Weinberg JM (2003) An overview of infliximab, etanercept, efalizumab, and alefacept as biologic therapy for psoriasis. *Clin Ther* 25: 2487–2505
4 Gottlieb AB, Evans R, Li S, Dooley LT, Guzzo CA, Baker D, Bala M, Marano CW, Menter A (2004) Infliximab induction therapy for patients with severe plaque-type psoriasis: a randomized,

double-blind, placebo-controlled trial. *J Am Acad Dermatol* 51: 534–542
5 Reich K, Nestle FO, Papp K, Ortonne JP, Evans R, Guzzo C, Li S, Dooley LT, Griffiths CE; EXPRESS study investigators (2005) Infliximab induction and maintenance therapy for moderate-to-severe psoriasis: a phase III, multicentre, double-blind trial. *Lancet* 366: 1367–1374
6 Leonardi C, Powers JL, Matheson RT, Goffe BS, Zitnik R, Wang A, Gottlieb AB; Etanercept Psoriasis Study Group (2003) Etanercept as monotherapy in patients with psoriasis. *N Engl J Med* 349: 2014–2022
7 Papp KA, Tyring S, Lahfa M, Prinz J, Griffiths CE, Nakanishi AM, Zitnik R, van de Kerkhof PC, Melvin L; Etanercept Psoriasis Study Group (2005) A global phase III randomized controlled trial of etanercept in psoriasis: safety, efficacy, and effect of dose reduction. *Br J Dermatol* 152: 1304–1312
8 Magliocco MA, Gottlieb AB (2004) Etanercept therapy for patients with psoriatic arthritis and concurrent hepatitis C virus infection: report of 3 cases. *J Am Acad Dermatol* 51: 580–584
9 (2003) Adalimumab (HUMIRA) for rheumatoid arthritis. *Med Lett Drugs Ther* 45: 25–27
10 Gordon KB, Leonardi C, Menter MA, Langley R, Chen DM (2004) Adalimumab efficacy and safety in patients with moderate to severe chronic plaque psoriasis: preliminary findings from a 12-week dose-ranging trial. Poster presented at: American Academy of Dermatology, 62nd Annual Meeting, Washington, DC, 6–11 February 2004, Poster 2
11 Langley R, Leonardi C, Toth D, Hoofman R (2005) Long-term safety and efficacy of adalimumab in the treatment of moderate to severe chronic plaque psoriasis. Poster presented at: 63rd Annual Meeting of the American Academy of Dermatology; 18–22 February 2005; New Orleans, LA, Poster 8
12 Lebwohl M (2002) New developments in the treatment of psoriasis. *Arch Dermatol* 138: 686–688
13 Keane J, Gershon S, Wise RP, Mirabile-Levens E, Kasznica J, Schwieterman WD, Siegel JN, Braun MM (2001) Tuberculosis associated with infliximab, a tumor necrosis factor alpha-neutralizing agent. *N Engl J Med* 345: 1098–1104 Bresnihan B, Cunnane G (2003) Infection complications associated with the use of biologic agents. *Rheum Dis Clin North Am* 29: 185–202
14 Gardam MA, Keystone EC, Menzies R, Manners S, Skamene E, Long R, Vinh DC (2003) Anti-tumour necrosis factor agents and tuberculosis risk: mechanisms of action and clinical management. *Lancet Infect Dis* 3: 148–155
15 Hamilton CD (2004) Infectious complications of treatment with biologic agents. *Curr Opin Rheumatol* 16: 393–398
16 Brown SL, Greene MH, Gershon SK, Edwards ET, Braun MM (2002) Tumor necrosis factor antagonist therapy and lymphoma development: twenty-six cases reported to the Food and Drug Administration. *Arthritis Rheum* 46: 3151–3158
17 Wolfe F, Michaud K (2004) Lymphoma in rheumatoid arthritis: the effect of methotrexate and anti-tumor necrosis factor therapy in 18'572 patients. *Arthritis Rheum* 50: 1740–1751
18 Adams AE, Zwicker J, Curiel C, Kadin ME, Falchuk KR, Drews R, Kupper TS (2004) Aggressive cutaneous T-cell lymphomas after TNF alpha blockade. *J Am Acad Dermatol* 51: 660–662
19 Wed MD (2005) Available at: http://my.webmd.com/content/article/95/103188.htm. Accessed 11 September 2005
20 FDA Advisory Committee (2005) Arthritis Committee. Will discuss risk of lymphoma with TNF inhibitors at March 4 meeting. Available at: http://www.fdaadvisorycommittee.com/FDC/AdvisoryCommittee/Committees/Arthritis±Drugs/030403_TNFsafety/030403_TNFsafetyP.htm. Accessed 11 September 2005
21 Mohan N, Edwards ET, Cupps TR, Oliverio PJ, Sandberg G, Crayton H, Richert JR, Siegel JN (2001) Demyelination occurring during anti-tumor necrosis factor alpha therapy for inflammatory arthritides. *Arthritis Rheum* 44: 2862–2869
22 Kwon HJ, Cote TR, Cuffe MS, Kramer JM, Braun MM (2003) Case reports of heart failure after therapy with a tumor necrosis factor antagonist. *Ann Intern Med* 138: 807–811
23 Debandt M, Vittecoq O, Descamps V, Le Loet X, Meyer O (2003) Anti-TNF-alpha-induced systemic lupus syndrome. *Clin Rheumatol* 22: 56–61
24 Watts RA (2000) Musculoskeletal and systemic reactions to biological therapeutic agents. *Curr Opin Rheumatol* 12: 49–52
25 Maini R, St Clair EW, Breedveld F, Furst D, Kalden J, Weisman M, Smolen J, Emery P, Harriman G, Feldmann M et al. (1999) Infliximab (chimeric anti-tumour necrosis factor alpha monoclonal antibody) *versus* placebo in rheumatoid arthritis patients receiving concomitant methotrexate: a randomised phase III trial. ATTRACT Study Group. *Lancet* 354: 1932–1939

26 Rutgeerts P, D'Haens G, Targan S, Vasiliauskas E, Hanauer SB, Present DH, Mayer L, Van Hogezand RA, Braakman T, DeWoody KL et al. (1999) Efficacy and safety of retreatment with anti-tumor necrosis factor antibody (infliximab) to maintain remission in Crohn's disease. *Gastroenterology* 117: 761–769
27 Shakoor N, Michalska M, Harris CA, Block JA (2002) Drug-induced systemic lupus erythematosus associated with etanercept therapy [letter]. *Lancet* 359: 579–580
28 Lebwohl M, Tyring SK, Hamilton TK, Toth D, Glazer S, Tawfik NH, Walicke P, Dummer W, Wang X, Garovoy MR et al. (2003) A novel targeted T-cell modulator, efalizumab, for plaque psoriasis. *N Engl J Med* 349: 2004–2013
29 Gordon KB, Papp KA, Hamilton TK, Walicke PA, Dummer W, Li N, Bresnahan BW, Menter A; Efalizumab Study Group (2003) Efalizumab for patients with moderate to severe plaque psoriasis: a randomized controlled trial. *JAMA* 290: 3073–3080
30 Menter A, Kardatzke D, Rundle AC, Kwon P, Garovoy MR, Leonardi CL (2004) Incidence and prevention of rebound upon efalizumab discontinuation. Poster presented at: 10th International Psoriasis Symposium, Toronto, Canada, 10–13 June 2004
31 Toth DP, Papp KA (2004) Managing recurrence of psoriasis following abrupt withdrawal form efalizumab therapy. Poster presented at: 10th International Psoriasis Symposium, Toronto, Canada, 10–13 June 2004
32 Cather JC, Menter A (2005) Efalizumab: continuous therapy for chronic psoriasis. *Expert Opin Biol Ther* 5: 393–403
33 Lebwohl M (2002) New developments in the treatment of psoriasis. *Arch Dermatol* 138: 686–688
34 RAPTIVA® (efalizumab) package insert. South San Francisco, Calif: Genentech, Inc; 2005
35 Lebwohl M, Christophers E, Langley R, Ortonne JP, Roberts J, Griffiths CE, Alefacept Clinical Study Group (2003) An international, randomized, double-blind, placebo-controlled phase 3 trial of intramuscular alefacept in patients with chronic plaque psoriasis. *Arch Dermatol* 139: 719–727
36 Krueger GG, Ellis CN (2003) Alefacept therapy produces remission for patients with chronic plaque psoriasis. *Br J Dermatol* 148: 784–788
37 Ellis CN, Krueger GG (2001) Treatment of chronic plaque psoriasis by selective targeting of memory effector T lymphocytes. *N Engl J Med* 345: 248–255
38 Gribetz CH, Blum R, Brady C, Cohen S, Lebwohl M (2004) Safety and efficacy of an extended course (16 weeks) of alefacept in the treatment of chronic plaque psoriasis. Poster presented at: Summer Academy 2004 of the American Academy of Dermatology; 28 July–1 August 2004; New York, Poster 74
39 AMEVIVE® (alefacept package insert). Cambridge, Mass: Biogen, Inc; 2005

Treatment of Psoriasis
Edited by J.M. Weinberg

Biologic and oral therapies in development for the treatment of psoriasis

Maria R. Robinson and Neil J. Korman

Department of Dermatology, Murdough Family Center for Psoriasis, University Hospitals Case Medical Center, Cleveland, OH 44106, USA

Introduction

Over the last several years, tremendous advances have been made in understanding the pathogenesis of psoriasis. These new insights have provided the framework for the development of several new classes of targeted therapies, including monoclonal antibodies and fusion proteins. Several of these drugs, including those targeting tumor necrosis factor and T cell activation, appear to be safe and effective over the short-term for the treatment of patients with psoriasis. As more is learned about the pathogenesis of psoriasis, novel therapeutic targets will be identified. It is the hope that these discoveries will continually develop into new therapies thus providing patients with psoriasis more effective treatment options. Here, we will briefly review new psoriasis therapies which are currently in development.

Small molecule targets

Calcineurin inhibitors

Calcineurin inhibitors (CNi) are effective in the treatment of psoriasis. Cyclosporine (CSA) is one of the most studied CNis and has been used to treat psoriasis for more than a decade. Cyclosporine forms a complex with cyclophilin, which inhibits calcineurin phosphatase and subsequently downregulates the transcription of a number of cytokine genes, most notably interleukin (IL)-2, which is a major T cell activator in psoriasis [1]. CSA is associated with significant toxicity, including nephrotoxicity and hypertension. Nephrotoxicity is dose-dependent and occurs at a higher frequency with prolonged use, both of which limit the use of cyclosporine to the short-term.

ISA247 is a novel oral CNi with a similar pharmacokinetic profile to CSA. It differs in the addition of a modified functional group on the amino acid 1 residue [2] and has been shown to be more potent than CSA in both *in vitro* and nonhuman primate studies [3–6]. In rabbits, ISA247 was associated with less renal toxicity, measured by creatinine clearance and renal histological changes, than CSA at comparable drug exposure [3].

ISA247 has been evaluated for the treatment of psoriasis in a Phase II, randomized, placebo-controlled trial [2]. A total of 201 patients were randomized in a 1:2:2 ratio to receive placebo, ISA247 1.0 mg/kg/d, or 3.0 mg/kg/d. Early in the study, three patients in the 3.0 mg/kg/d group experienced elevated creatinine levels, and so the dosing levels were adjusted to placebo, ISA247 0.5 mg/kg/d, or 1.5 mg/kg/d. By the fourth week, a significant proportion of patients had a 75% improvement in their PASI scores in the treatment groups *versus* the placebo group (0.0% placebo, 4.5% 0.5 mg/kg, and 26.5% 1.5 mg/kg/d, $p = 0.013$). In the 1.5 mg/kg group, there was a statistically significant increase in mean creatinine levels over baseline, though all the levels remained within the normal range. Notably, the nine patients who demonstrated a 30% rise in serum creatinine were all being treated with potentially nephrotoxic drugs.

Because ISA247 has demonstrated increased potency and fewer toxicities than CSA, it may be a promising option for the treatment of psoriasis. More clinical trials are needed to further evaluate the potential value of ISA247 in the treatment of psoriasis.

Fumaric acid

Fumaric acid esters (FAEs) have shown to be effective in the treatment of psoriasis [7, 8] and a defined mixture of FAEs was approved in Germany in 1994 [9].

Dimethylfumarate (DMF) is rapidly hydrolyzed to monomethylfumarate (MMF), which is thought to be the active compound in fumaric acid esters [10]. FAEs are thought to inhibit T cell activity partially through apoptosis of activated T cells [11] and through a shift from a T-helper (Th)1-type response to a Th2-type response, thus inhibiting the key Th1 cytokines IL-2, IL-12 and interferon-γ [9]. The use of FAEs has been limited by their toxicities, including gastrointestinal complaints and flushing, which occur in up to 60% and 30% of patients, respectively [9].

A novel, second-generation, oral fumaric acid derivative, BG-12, has been developed in an effort to reduce the toxicities associated with the currently available FAEs. In a Phase II double-blind, placebo-controlled trial, 144 patients were randomized to receive one of four treatments: placebo or BG-12 (120, 360, or 720 mg/day). At 12 weeks, 42% of patients in the 720 mg/day group reached a 75% improvement in their PASI (Psoriasis and Severity Index) Score compared to 11% in the placebo group [12]. BG-12 was well tolerated. Common adverse events were mild-to-moderate in severity, and included flushing, upper respiratory infections, and elevated liver function tests [12]. In a Phase III study, 175 patients with psoriasis were randomized 3:2 to receive

720 mg/day BG-12 or placebo. At week 16, the median PASI score was significantly lower in the BG-12 group compared with the placebo (5.8 *versus* 14.2, $P < 0.001$) [12, 13]. Adverse events were mild-to-moderate in severity and flushing was the most common event (42% *versus* 9%) [13]. These results suggest that BG12 could prove to be a valuable oral therapeutic option for the treatment of psoriasis; further studies are warranted.

Phosphodiesterase inhibitor

Phosphodiesterase (PDE) 4 is an enzyme important in the signaling associated with the inflammatory process, and CC-10004 is an oral PDE4 inhibitor that downregulates the transcription of proinflammatory cytokines [14]. In an open label, single-arm Phase II study for psoriasis, 20 mg of CC-10004 was given to 17 patients once daily for 29 days [15]. An interim study analysis of nine patients demonstrated that CC-10004 was associated with a decrease in epidermal thickness and decreases in epidermal and dermal inflammation of psoriatic plaques. Further studies are needed to asses CC-10004 as a potential treatment for psoriasis.

Cytokine targets

TNF antagonists

Neutralization of tumor necrosis factor alpha (TNF) has proven to be a safe and efficacious treatment for psoriasis. Two TNF inhibitors, etanercept and infliximab, are currently FDA approved for the treatment of moderate to severe plaque psoriasis. Etanercept is a recombinant human p75 soluble TNF receptor comprised of two TNF-α binding domains linked to the Fc portion of human Ig. Infliximab is a chimeric monoclonal antibody comprised of a human Ig Fc portion and a murine TNF-α binding variable region. Adalimumab, a fully human recombinant IgG monoclonal antibody, is a third TNF antagonist that is in late stage clinical investigation for the treatment of psoriasis. A Phase II double-blind, placebo controlled study of 147 patients demonstrated that adalimumab was efficacious and well-tolerated [16].

A novel TNF antagonist, certolizumab, is currently under investigation for the treatment of several immunologically mediated diseases, including rheumatoid arthritis, Crohn's disease, and psoriasis. Certolizumab is an engineered human anti-TNF-α Fab fragment linked to polyethylene glycol (PEG). The addition of a PEG moiety increases the plasma half-life to almost 14 days thereby permitting less frequent dosing [17]. In Phase I and II clinical studies for rheumatoid arthritis and Crohn's disease, certolizumab was shown to be effective and well-tolerated [17–20]. Certolizumab has also shown promising results in the treatment of psoriasis. In a Phase II study, 176 patients were randomized to receive placebo or one of two dosing regimens of certolizumab: 200 mg or 400 mg every other week after an initial dose of 400 mg. By week 12, significantly more patients in the certolizumab groups achieved a 75% reduction from baseline in PASI score when compared to placebo (placebo: 6.8%, 200 mg: 74.6%, 400 mg: 82.8% ($p < 0.001$)) [21].

Interleukin-12 and interleukin-23

Interleukins (IL)-12 and -23 are critical regulatory cytokines involved in the pathogenesis of psoriasis and thus serve as another potential therapeutic target. IL-12 plays a very important role in the proliferation and activation of T cells and helps produce a T-helper (Th)-1 response. IL-23 promotes the development of Th17 cells resulting in proliferation and activation of macrophages. IL-12 and IL-23 are both heterodimers and share a common subunit, p40, whose expression is upregulated in psoriatic plaques [22, 23].

Early clinical studies evaluating anti-IL-12/23 (anti-IL12p40) as a treatment for psoriasis have shown promising results. The first open label Phase I trial demonstrated that one dose of intravenous (IV) anti-IL-12/23 resulted in dramatic improvement in psoriasis in the majority of patients [24]. A double-blind, placebo-controlled Phase I trial later showed that subcutaneous (SQ) anti-IL-12/23 was comparable to the IV formulation [25].

In a Phase II, double-blind, placebo-controlled clinical trial, 320 patients were randomized to receive placebo or one of four treatment regimens with SQ CNTO 1275 (1 dose of 45 mg or 90 mg, 4 weekly injections with 45 mg or 90 mg [26]. By week 12, a 75% improvement in baseline PASI scores was observed in 52%, 59%, 67%, or 81% of the patients treated with 45 mg, 90 mg, 4 weekly 45 mg injections, or 4 weekly 90 mg injections, respectively, compared to only 2% in the placebo group ($p < 0.001$ for each comparison). Overall, CNTO 1275 was well tolerated and serious adverse events were uncommon in all groups [26].

STA-5326, an oral IL-12/23 inhibitor, has been studied in patients with psoriasis [27].

Other targets

Anti-CD80

T cell activation requires at least two signals from antigen-presenting cells (APCs). The primary signal is mediated through the interaction between the T cell receptor and a specific antigen bound to the major histocompatibility complex (MHC). The second signal is antigen-independent and is mediated by co-stimulatory signals, including CD80 (B7-1) and CD86 (B7-2) on antigen-presenting cells (APC). Both CD80 and CD86 each bind to CD28 on T cells to promote T cell activation. CD152, which is expressed by activated T cells, can also bind to CD80 and CD86 and results in downregulation of T cell responses [28].

Galiximab is an IgG anti-CD80 monoclonal antibody which blocks the CD80–CD28 interaction, but not the CD80–CD152 interaction. In Phase I and II trials for psoriasis, galiximab showed preliminary evidence of efficacy, however the most appropriate dosing regimen was not ascertained [28, 29]. Further evaluation of this agent will be necessary to determine its effectiveness as a potential treatment for psoriasis.

Conclusion

Targeted immunotherapeutics are a valuable new treatment option for patients with moderate to severe psoriasis. Modern science and advanced immunologic techniques have replaced serendipity in the discovery of these new therapies. While short-term data suggest that these drugs are safe, more time is needed to assess adequately their safety. If it is demonstrated that these therapies have greater safety and efficacy profiles when compared to traditional therapies, they will likely become first line agents. In order to best serve their patients, clinicians should continually be knowledgeable of new treatment options for psoriasis.

References

1 Ho VC (2004) The use of ciclosporin in psoriasis: a clinical review. *Br J Dermatol* 150: 1–10

2 Bissonnette R, Papp K, Poulin Y, Lauzon G, Aspeslet L, Huizinga R, Mayo P, Foster RT, Yatscoff RW, Maksymowych WP (2006) A randomized, multicenter, double-blind, placebo-controlled phase 2 trial of ISA247 in patients with chronic plaque psoriasis. *J Am Acad Dermatol* 54: 472–478

3 Aspeslet L, Freitag D, Trepanier D, Abel M, Naicker S, Kneteman N, Foster R, Yatscoff R (2001) $ISA_{TX}247$: a novel calcineurin inhibitor. *Transplantation Proceedings* 33: 1048–1051

4 Birsan T, Dambrin C, Freitag DG, Yatscoff RW, Morris RE (2005) The novel calcineurin inhibitor ISA247: a more potent immunosuppressant than cyclosporine *in vitro*. *Transpl Int* 17: 767–771

5 Stalder M, Birsan T, Hubble RW, Paniagua RT, Morris RE (2003) *In vivo* evaluation of the novel calcineurin inhibitor $ISA_{TX}247$ non-human primates. *J Heart Lung Transplant* 22: 1343–1352

6 Gregory CR, Kyles AE, Bernsteen L, Wagner GS, Tarantal AF, Christe KL, Brignolo L, Spinner A, Griffey SM, Paniagua RT et al. (2004) Compared with cyclosporine, $ISA_{TX}247$ significantly prolongs renal-allograft survival in a nonhuman primate model. *Transplantation* 78: 681–685

7 Nugteren-Huying WM, van der Schroeff JG, Hermans J, Suurmond D (1990) Fumaric acid therapy for psoriasis: a randomized, double-blind, placebo-controlled study. *J Am Acad Dermatol* 22: 311–312

8 Altmeyer PJ, Matthes U, Pawlak F, Hoffmann K, Frosch PJ, Ruppert P, Wassilew SW, Horn T, Kreysel HW, Lutz G et al. (1994) Antipsoriatic effect of fumaric acid derivatives. Results of a multicenter double-blind study in 100 patients. *J Am Acad Dermatol* 30: 977–981

9 Ormerod AD, Mrowietz U (2004) Fumaric acid esters, their place in the treatment of psoriasis. *Br J Dermatol* 150: 630–632

10 Mrowietz U, Christophers E, Altmeyer P (1999) Treatment of severe psoriasis with fumaric acid esters: scientific background and guidelines for therapeutic use. *Br J Dermatol* 141: 424–429

11 Treumer F, Zhu K, Glaser R, Mrowietz U (2003) Dimethylfumarate is a potent inducer of apoptosis in human T cells. *J Invest Dermatol* 121: 1383–1388

12 (2005) BG 12: BG 00012, BG 12/Oral Fumarate, FAG-201, second-generation fumarate derivative – Fumapharm/Biogen Idec. *Drugs R D* 6: 229–230
13 Mrowietz U, Reich K, Spellman MC (2006) Efficacy, safety, and quality of life effects of a novel oral formulation of dimethyl fumarate in patients with moderate to severe plaque psoriasis: results of a phase 3 study. *J Am Acad Derm* 54, no 3, Supp Mar 2006: AB202, P2816
14 Khobzaoui M, Gutke HJ, Burnet M (2005) CC-10004. *Curr Opin Invst Drugs* 6: 518–525
15 Gottlieb AB, Malaviya R, Rohane P, Jones M (2006) Biological activity of CC-10004 with severe plaque-type psoriasis. *J Am Acad Dermatol* 54, no 3, Supp Mar 2006: AB9, P34
16 Gordon KB, Langley RG, Leonardi C, Toth D, Menter MA, Kang S, Heffernan M, Miller B, Hamlin R, Lim L et al. (2006) Clinical response to adalimumab treatment in patients with moderate to severe psoriasis: double-blind, randomized controlled trial and open-label extension study. *J Am Acad Derm* 55: 598–606
17 Kaushik VV, Moots RJ (2005) CDP-870 (certolizumab) in rheumatoid arthritis. *Expert Opin Biol Ther* 5: 601–606
18 Choy EH, Hazleman B, Smith M, Moss K, Lisi L, Scott DG, Patel J, Sopwith M, Isenberg DA (2002) Efficacy of a novel PEGylated humanized anti-TNF fragment (CDP870) in patients with rheumatoid arthritis: a phase II double-blinded, randomized, dose-escalating trial. *Rheumatology* 41: 1133–1137
19 Winter TA, Wright J, Ghosh S, Jahnsens J, Innes A, Round P (2004) Intravenous CDP870, a PEGylated Fab_ fragment of a humanized antitumour necrosis factor antibody, in patients with moderate-to-severe Crohn's disease: an exploratory study. *Aliment Pharmacol Ther* 20: 1337–1346
20 Schreiber S, Rutgeerts P, Fedorak RN, Khaliq-Kareemi M, Kamm MA, Boivin M, Bernstein CN, Staun M, Thomsen O, Innes A (2005) A randomized, placebo-controlled trial of certolizumab pegol (CDP870) for treatment of Crohn's disease. *Gastroenterology* 129: 807–818
21 Ortonne JP, Sterry W, Tasset C, Reich K (2007) Efficacy and safety of subcutaneous certolizumab pegol, the first PEGylated anti-TNFα, in patients with moderate-to-severe chronic plaque psoriasis: preliminary results from a double-blind, placebo-controlled trial. *J Am Acad Derm* 56, Supp2, Feb 2007: AB6, P21
22 Park H, Li Z, Yang XO, Chang SH, Nurieva R, Wang YH, Wang Y, Hood L, Zhu Z, Tian Q et al. (2005) A distinct lineage of CD4 T cells regulates tissue inflammation by producing interleukin 17. *Nat Immunol* 6: 1133–1141
23 Yawalkar N, Karlen S, Hunger R, Brand CU, Braathen LR (1998) Expression of interleukin-12 is increased in psoriatic skin. *J Invest Dermatol* 111: 1053–1057
24 Kauffman CL, Aria N, Toichi E, McCormick TS, Cooper KD, Gottlieb AB, Everitt DE, Frederick B, Zhu Y, Graham MA et al. (2004) A phase I study evaluating the safety, pharmacokinetics, and clinical response of a human IL-12 p40 antibody in subjects with plaque psoriasis. *J Invest Dermatol* 123: 1037–1044
25 Gottlieb A, Frederick B, Everitt D, McCormick T (2005) A phase 1 study evaluating the safety, pharmacokinetics, and clinical response of a human IL-12 P40 antibody administered subcutaneously in subjects with plaque psoriasis. *J Am Acad Dermato* 52, part 2, No 3: p.172, p.2705
26 Krueger GG, Langely RG, Leonardi C, Yeilding N, Guzzo C, Wang Y, Dooley LT, Lebwohl M (2007) A human interleukin-12/23 monoclonal antibody for the treatment of psoriasis. *N Engl J Med* 356: 580–592
27 Gottlieb A, Cather J, Hamilton T, Sherman M (2006) Preliminary clinical safety and efficacy results from an open-label phase 2 study of STA-5326, an oral IL-12/IL-23 inhibitor, in patients with moderate to severe chronic plaque psoriasis. *J Am Acad Dermatol* 54, Suppl no3, Mar 2006: AB10, p.37
28 Gottlieb AB, Kang S, Linden KG, Lebwohl M, Menter A, Abdulghani AA, Goldfarb M, Chieffo N, Totoritis MC (2004) Evaluation of safety and clinical activity of multiple doses of the anti-CD80 monoclonal antibody, galiximab, in patients with moderate to severe plaque psoriasis. *Clin Immunolog* 111: 28–37
29 Gottlieb AB, Lebwohl M, Totoritis MC, Abdulghani AA, Sheuy SR, Romano P, Chaudhari U, Allen RS, Lizambri RG (2002) Clinical and histologic response to single-dose treatment of moderate to severe psoriasis with an anti-CD80 monoclonal antibody. *J Am Acad Dermatol* 47: 692–700

Treatment of Psoriasis
Edited by J.M. Weinberg

Quality of life issues in psoriasis

Amanda B. Sergay, Matthew Silvan and Jeffrey M. Weinberg

Department of Dermatology, St. Luke's-Roosevelt Hospital Center and Beth Israel Medical Center, New York, NY, USA

Introduction

Health-related quality of life (HRQOL), has been defined as "peoples' subjective evaluation of the influences of their current health status… on their ability to achieve and maintain a level of overall functioning that allows them to pursue valued life goals and that is reflected in general wellbeing" [1, 2]. Psoriasis is a chronic disease with physical, psychosocial, and economic implications that commonly interfere with patients' daily functional capacity, and consequently, their quality of life.

In 2006, the National Psoriasis Foundation surveyed over 500 patients and found that 80% of respondents with psoriasis and 85% of patients with psoriatic arthritis considered their disease to be a moderate to large problem in their lives [3]. Many healthcare professionals base their clinical assessment on physical signs and symptoms, and by using conventional measures such as the Psoriasis Area and Severity Index (PASI) score. However, clinical severity of psoriasis is not always an accurate predictor of the extent to which psoriasis affects a patient's quality of life. Studies have shown that the PASI score does not always correlate with patients' assessments of their quality of life, nor does it provide a full indication of the psychosocial disability they face [4, 5]. In fact, a patient's perceived severity of psoriasis has been shown to be related to the distress they feel on a daily basis [6]. Since psoriasis can affect some patients with mild disease to the same degree as those with very severe disease, it is necessary to evaluate the physical manifestations and the psoriasis-related quality of life when assessing the disease's overall impact.

Quality of life measures

In order to accurately assess HRQOL, many measures have been developed and utilized in clinical studies. In addition to general quality of life measures, dermatology-specific and psoriasis-specific instruments have been created that provide more defined information about how skin diseases affect patients on various physical and psychosocial dimensions. While a detailed description of the differences between these indices is beyond the scope of this chapter, it is important to be aware of these measures because they are the foundation for much of the quality of life data in the literature. Underscoring their importance, forums such as the Group for Research and Assessment of Psoriasis and Psoriatic Arthritis and the International Psoriasis Council have recently been created to ensure the validity and standardization of these instruments [7]. General measures of quality of life include HAQ (Health Assessment Questionnaire) and the SF-36 (Short-Form 36). Dermatology-specific measures include the DLQI (Dermatology Life Quality Index), DQOLS (Dermatology Quality of Life Scale), and the Skindex-29. The DLQI is the most utilized and validated measure of HRQOL in psoriasis and it is calculated from a summary of ten items that measure six subscales: symptoms and feelings, daily activities, leisure, work and school, personal relationships, and treatment satisfaction [7, 8]. Psoriasis-specific measures include IPSO (Impact of Psoriasis Questionnaire), KMPI (Koo-Menter Psoriasis Instrument), PDI (Psoriasis Disability Index), PLSI (Psoriasis Life Stress Inventory), and SPI (Salford Psoriasis Index.) The large number of instruments available reflects the multitude of dimensions that are involved in evaluating quality of life; patient evaluations often warrant the use of multiple instruments in order to ensure adequate assessment.

Physical impact

The cutaneous and arthritic manifestations of psoriasis can significantly impact the physical capabilities of patients. This physical impairment has been shown to be comparable to patients with other chronic diseases such as cancer, heart disease, hypertension, diabetes, arthritis and depression [1, 9]. The National Psoriasis Foundation (NPF) sponsored a large survey in 1998 and found that 26% of psoriasis patients claim their disease forced them to alter or stop their normal day-to-day activities [10]. In the 2005 NPF Survey Panel, 36% reported problems using their hands, 31% had problems walking, 31% had problems sitting and 31% had problems standing for long periods of time in the past month due to their psoriasis [11]. EUROPSO (European Federation of Psoriasis Patient Associations) surveyed 17'990 psoriasis patients and found that the greatest impact on quality of life centered around activities of daily living, especially activities related to physical appearance [12]. Such activities include clothing choice and participating in physical activities that may cause sweating or increased visibility. The respondents with moderate or severe disease were most affected, but patients with mild surface involvement were affected as well [12]. Interestingly, the only time direct correlations between PASI scores and quality of life are demonstrated, occurs when psoriasis affects areas of the body that are visible [6]. Patients may be more reticent to involve themselves in physical activities in which the lesions will be seen, such as swimming or sexual activity. Illustrating this point 26% of patients reported the disease interfered with their sexual activities in the past month [12].

Such physical impairments have the greatest impact in elderly psoriasis patients. The 1998 NPF survey found that elderly patients, 55 years of age and older, had the greatest physical impairments and were more likely to report difficulties in activities of daily living [10]. These restrictions are further impacted by psoriatic arthritis, the prevalence of which increases with age [13]. Psoriatic arthritis, in elderly and non-elderly patients, commonly affects the digits, the spine and back, and the insertion sites between tendons and ligaments [7, 14]. Physical mobility becomes extremely limited when inflammation of these joints leads to swelling and pain [5].

Physical impairment can vary with site of involvement. In particular, nail involvement and palmoplantar disease has been shown to restrict daily activities [9, 15, 16]. Psoriasis has also been shown to compromise the patient's ability to sleep well. In the 2005 NPF survey panel, nearly one half (48%) of respondents reported problems sleeping in the past month due to their psoriasis [11]. While the sleep disturbance may be related to physical discomfort, it also may be a psychological manifestation. (The psychosocial manifestations of psoriasis will be discusses later in the chapter.) Regardless, when sleep is disturbed, the physical functioning status, and likely job performance, can be negatively affected.

This negative impact of psoriasis on the workplace has been well documented. In the NPF survey panel from the third quarter of 2004, 26% of psoriasis patients and 48% of patients with psoriatic arthritis reported psoriasis negatively affected their job. 74% of respondents reported missing days from work for treatment of psoriasis and/or psoriatic arthritis [17]. Not surprisingly, a direct correlation between a reduction in work productivity and psoriasis severity has been shown [18]. A study by Finlay et al., found that out of 369 patients with severe psoriasis, one-third of those not working attributed this to psoriasis, and they found working patients missed an average of 26 days a year directly related to their psoriasis [19]. Many feel that any type of intervention that would improve the patients' quality of life could reduce psoriasis related productivity loss [20].

Besides decreased work productivity, the financial burden of psoriasis also comes from chronic and expensive treatment modalities. In 1998, annual outpatient costs were estimated to range from $1'400 to $6'600 per patient [21]. However, these estimates were calculated before the more costly biologic therapies and narrowband UVB therapy became more prevalent, so today's estimates would likely be even higher. In addition to prescription pharmaceuticals, many patients use over-the-counter treatments. The EUROPSO survey found that while 77% of patients had tried prescription modalities, the current use was low (40%), and 37% were using over-the-counter medication or treatment and 8.4% were using some form of thermal spa treatment [12]. Thus, when making decisions about treatment in psoriasis, the total cost to the patient must be seen as not only the cost of treating, but also the cost of not treating.

Psychosocial impact

Many patients consider stress to play a prominent role in their disease, but it is uncertain whether stress is a precipitant or consequence of psoriasis. It is clear, though, that psoriasis is associated with significant psychological morbidity and social anguish [22]. Although studies vary, about one in four psoriasis patients experience significant psychological distress [23]. Patients with psoriasis have been shown to have a higher rate of depression and suicidal tendencies than non-psoriatic subjects [7, 22, 24]. In a study of over 2'000 Italian patients with psoriasis depression was noted in 62% [22]. A significantly higher proportion of women exhibited depressive symptomatology, but interestingly, men aged 40 and younger were significantly more likely to report depressive symptoms than men older than 40. In addition, patients with a university level education were significantly less likely to report depressive symptoms [22]. While it is agreed that the primary predictor of depression in these patients is the clinical severity of their psoriasis, symptoms such as pruritus and feelings of stigma that arise from the deprivation of social touch have also shown to be related to depression, as well [9, 25–27].

Similarly, many studies have found higher levels of anxiety and excessive worry in patients with psoriasis when compared with controls [9, 28]. Hypervigilance about a social threat followed by its avoidance is felt to accompany and maintain the anxiety experienced by these patients [9]. Other studies have found anticipation and avoidant coping behaviors to be significantly associated with disability [9, 29, 30]. While excessive worry can cause distress to the patient, it has also been shown to negatively impact treatment outcomes. Fortune et al. showed that patients who qualify as 'high level' worriers according to the PSWQ (Penn State Worry Questionnaire) cleared with psoralen-UVA (PUVA) treatment 1.8 times slower than that of the low-level worriers [31].

Data from the 2006 Spring NPF survey, underscores the psychosocial impact of psoriasis: 48% of respondents reported strong feelings of anger and frustration, 40% reported feeling helpless and 38% reported self-consciousness. 29% of respondents reported explaining their psoriasis to others between one and three times per week, while 11% explain their disease at least once a day. Patients with more severe psoriasis reported explaining their disease to others more often [3]. More than half the respondents in the 1998 NPF survey (54%) reported experiencing life disruptions and social withdrawal as a result of their psoriasis [7, 10].

Studies have showed that one of the primary predictors of disability in psoriasis patients is the perception of stigmatization [9, 28, 32]. It is also thought that this perception accounts for much of the variations in disability among psoriatic patients [9]. An example of this sense of stigmatization was seen in the 1998 NPF survey in which 40% have reported experiencing problems with receiving equal service in service establishments [10]. Social stress from others' reactions to psoriatic lesions have been shown to impact patient disability scores more negatively than any other variable including disease severity and duration of disease [29].

Naturally, psychosocial distress negatively impacts a patient's quality of life. One study showed that dermatologists commonly underestimate the prevalence of psychiatric morbidity among their patients [22, 33]. In order to properly evaluate the severity of psoriasis, healthcare professionals must take into account its psychosocial impact.

Social and demographic variables

There is conflicting data in the literature concerning the impact that age has on psoriasis. Many studies have found that the impact of psoriasis decreases with increasing age [5, 34]. One supporting example was the previously discussed finding that psoriasis appears to have a greater psychological impact on younger men [22]. However, when teasing apart the components of quality of life, elderly patients have been shown to have more physical disability than younger patients, but less psychological distress [3, 10]. Other studies have found that older psoriasis patients (age > 65 years), regardless of severity, have a lower skin-related quality of life, not only in terms of physical health, but also psychosocially [35]. Even when controlling for factors such as depression and anxiety, (common problems in older patients) these patients still scored lower on the Skindex-29. Because the studies implemented different quality of life measurements and because it is impossible to generalize about any one population of patients, such conflicting data can be expected.

Several studies have shown women to report more impairment in skin-related quality of life when compared with men [35, 36]. One study found that women report a more pronounced feeling of discrimination [37]. Some hypothesize that this gender difference can be explained by the data showing that women are more focused on appearance and tend to be less satisfied with their body image [35]. In other studies, women with skin disease have been found to experience greater interference with their social and sex lives, and have more subjective stress and worry [4, 38]. In Zachariae's study of over 6'000 Nordic patients, women reported greater disease severity and affected area than men, but men had greater PASI scores [5]. However, when controlling for disease severity and other socio-economic and demographic variables, gender was not a predictor of quality of life. Similarly, Gupta and Gupta found no gender differences in quality of life measures related to appearance and socialization, but their male patients reported greater work-related stresses [34].

Marriage or living with a partner, having university level of education, and being employed have been shown to have significant beneficial effects on self-reported disease severity and quality of life [5, 39, 40]. A statistically significant association was seen between both impairment of psoriasis-related quality of life and disease severity, and alcohol consumption, cigarette smoking, and use of tranquilizers, sleeping pills and antidepressants. Because alcohol and smoking have been shown to be possible risk factors for psoriasis [5, 41] it is impossible to discern whether these associations are indicative of poor coping mechanisms and poor HRQOL, or are actual risk factors for the exacerbation of existing disease [5].

In an attempt to identify other factors that cause variability in the impact of psoriasis, Unaeze et al. performed a prospective study of 484 patients with psoriasis to examine the HRQOL of patients at baseline and over an 11 year time period. After adjusting for confounders, the significant predictors of baseline IPSO (Impact of Psoriasis Questionnaire) scores, included older age, poor general health, earlier age of psoriasis onset and higher numbers of prescription drugs. Interestingly, only self-reported general health was a significant predictor of change in IPSO score 11 years after baseline [42].

Treatment and quality of life

Although none of the treatments for psoriasis are curative, significant improvement in HRQOL has been observed with many of the available modalities. One study found that more than 50% physical clearance must be attained before meaningful change in quality of life is reported by patients [43].

Most of the studies examining HRQOL have evaluated the newer biologic therapies, so the data is somewhat limited in regard to older treatments such as phototherapy [7]. Etanercept (Enbrel), Alefacept (Amevive), and Efalizumab (Raptiva) were the three biologics that have been approved for psoriasis in the US. Many studies have shown biologic therapies to both alleviate the physical symptoms of psoriasis, and to improve patients' satisfaction with therapy and overall quality of life. However, few studies have performed head-to-head comparisons of these agents.

In a randomized, Phase III trial, patients with psoriasis received either placebo, etanercept 50 mg per week, or etanercept 50 mg twice weekly during a 12-week, double-blind period. The DLQI total score improved by a mean of 7.7–8.0 points at week 12, depending on etanercept dosage [44]. The DLQI subscales showing the greatest improvement with etanercept therapy were the symptoms and feelings subscale and daily activities subscale. Pruritus was assessed by having patients rate their itch on a scale of 0 (no itching) to 5 (severe itching.) Mean improvement of pruritus from baseline to week 12 was 0.5 points (1%) in the placebo group, 1.55 points (49%) in the etanercept 50 mg per week group, and 2.51 points (72%) in the etanercept 50 mg BIW group [44]. Significant improvement from baseline was also noted in the SF-36 general measure of HRQOL. Multiple studies have found that greater improvements in DLQI are achieved with increased time and dosage of etanercept [7, 45–47] and improvement in quality of life has been shown to occur as early as 2 weeks after the start treatment [48].

Alefacept has also been shown to improve the quality of life, as measured by the DLQI and DQOLS [7, 43, 49]. Feldman et al., showed that at 12 weeks after the last dose of alefacept, the mean change in DQOLS was 3.4 points compared with 1.4 points for placebo. However, mean changes in SF-36 scores were not significant between the treatment groups [49]. It is important to note that patients who use alefacept must see their doctor weekly for intramuscular injections and phlebotomy for CD4 counts. This may contribute to alefacept's lower efficacy in regard to quality of life improvement when compared with etanercept [7].

Efalizumab also improves DLQI scores when compared with placebo controls and has been shown to be somewhat superior to alefacept in this domain. The International Phase III Clinical Experience with Raptiva (CLEAR) trial evaluating the efficacy of efalizumab in patients with moderate to severe plaque psoriasis. While a significant improvement was seen by week 4, at week 12, patients receiving efalizumab had a significantly improved DLQI from baseline (5.7 points) compared with placebo controls (2.3 points). Patients also showed significant improvement compared with placebo in the SF-36 score. The severity of itching was also measured in this study using an itching scale with scores ranged from 0 (no itching) to 10 (severe itching). The mean itching score improved from baseline by 2.5 points at week 12 compared to 0.6 points for patients receiving placebo [7, 50].

Progress has also been shown with non-biologic therapy. Oral tazarotene, NBUVB, and leflunomide have been shown to significantly improve the HRQOL when compared with controls receiving a placebo [7, 51–53]. Intermittent short courses of cyclosporin and methotrexate were found to be equally effective [54–56]. Quality of life has also been evaluated in patients using topical treatments. For example, patients with mild to moderate plaque type psoriasis ranked Clobetasol foam (0.05%) as superior to other topical formulations (creams, lotions, ointments) based on factors impacting their quality of life [54, 56]. The study also showed that patients using the foam were more compliant. While quality of life and disease severity are improved with the more traditional, non-biologic therapies, many of these are associated with cumulative toxicity, inconvenience, and rapid relapse after treatment has been stopped [57]. Clearly, these aspects of treatment can significantly impact a patient's quality of life.

It is also important to assess patients' perspectives on their treatment when evaluating the overall impact of the disease on their lives. The treatment options in psoriasis are often inconvenient, messy and associated with side effects [58]. In a survey of over 18'000 psoriasis patients, almost three-quarters of respondents expressed low to moderate satisfaction with their treatment. 50% of patients reported that the most troubling aspect of therapy is its time consuming nature while 32% reported treatment ineffectiveness as the most troublesome aspect [12]. In the 2006 NPF survey, 29% of respondents report spending 30 min a day caring for their psoriasis, while 24% spends 60 min or more [3]. Dissatisfaction with treatment can lead to non-compliance, and consequently, treatment failure [6, 59].

What can we do?

Since psoriasis can have such a profound impact on physical and psychosocial aspects of patients' lives, the physician must integrate quality of life assessments with physical examinations in order to make appropriate treatment decisions. A study involving 238 dermatology outpatients was done to see if these quality of life assessments were being done. Quality of life discussions were absent in 40% of these patients' visits [60]. More quality of life discussions occurred with patients whose subsequent DLQI scores demonstrated a lower quality of life. The authors purport that clinicians may have felt they had a general sense of their patients' quality of life, and only brought the subject up with those patients they felt were most impacted by the disease. In addition, such patients likely initiated more quality of life discussions. Nonetheless, some patients with poor DLQI scores did not receive quality of life discussions. If quality of life measures were evaluated regularly with all patients, optimal, individualized care would more likely be delivered.

It has been shown that patient-centered visits that include quality of life discussions are associated with increased patient satisfaction, compliance with treatment, and symptom reduction with improved psychological status [60]. Patient-centered care refers to "health care that is closely congruent with and responsive to patients' wants, needs and preferences" [61]. Patient-centered care is especially helpful with psoriasis because optimal management requires patients' full involvement [61]. Implementing the patient-centered model includes educating the patient about the disease, providing realistic expectations for treatment, and paying attention to signs of psychological distress such as poor eye contact, flat affect or low energy levels. Also, involving patients in the decisions about treatment can help to give patients a sense of control [61]. Since perceived helplessness has been shown as the greatest predictor of stigmatization in psoriasis [9, 62], empowering patients with education and a sense of control may function to improve their quality of life.

While it is widely accepted that patients benefit from being well-educated about their disease, there are few studies that are demonstrative of this principle. In the Netherlands, a disease management program (consisting of psoriasis education, disease management training, and psychological support), together with topical treatment, was shown to improve disease severity and quality of life as measured by the skindex-29 [63]. Patients reported feeling emotionally stronger and felt more positively about living with psoriasis in the future.

Many patient advocacy groups share in this belief about patient education and aim to educate fellow patients about their disease and about treatments available to them. An example of such an advocacy group is the National Psoriasis Foundation (NPF.) The stated goal of the NPF is "to improve the quality of life of people who have psoriasis and psoriatic arthritis" [64, 65]. A study that evaluated the members of the NPF found that although members were significantly older and had more extensive disease, satisfaction with therapy was higher and disease burden was significantly lower as reported by members *versus* non-members [66]. This finding may suggest that disease education (enhanced by membership) can have benefits on psoriasis-related quality of life [64, 65]. Similarly, Jankowiak et al., examined the influence of patient education about psoriasis on their quality of life. With less information about their disease, patients had a lower quality of life index as measured by PDI (Psoriasis Disability Index) [67].

Although there is a lack of consensus in the literature, psychologic intervention such as cognitive and behavioral therapy, education and stress management procedures, or support alone has been shown to lead to clinical improvement in some psoriasis patients [68]. One example from Fortune et al., showed that cognitive behavior therapy as an adjunct to pharmacological therapy significantly improved the clinical severity of psoriasis during a 6 week course of treatment and for at least 6 months afterward [68]. Another study looked at the benefit of psychotherapy by having the psoriasis patients attend 90 min group therapy sessions weekly for 8 weeks. Their levels of anxiety were significantly reduced after the sessions at 6 month follow-up. Modest physical improvement in psoriasis severity was also seen [69]. A mindfulness meditation-based stress reduction audiotape during UV therapy was shown to increase the rate of skin clearing and decrease the number of sessions necessary to achieve clearing [70]. In addition, there are also a number of anecdotal reports of improvement in overall management of psoriasis with hypnosis, support groups, lessening psychosocial stressors, and psychotropic drugs [58, 71]. Accordingly, in addition to pharmacological intervention, it is clear the goal of treatment should aim to increase patients' feelings of control over their disease process, to encourage expression of emotions, and to educate about the disease.

Conclusions

It is not difficult to understand why a chronic, unpredictable, disfiguring disease that requires often unpleasant, long-term treatment, has the potential to adversely affect quality of life [71]. Psoriasis-related quality of life is a broad term that aims to incorporate with physical, psychosocial and economic implications and their cumulative impact on the patient. Each patient is an individual so the sum total of these dimensions differs from patient to patient. In turn, communication between the healthcare professional and the patient is paramount. Since higher rates of noncompliance and treatment failures are associated with poor communication and misunderstandings between the physician and the patient [72], discussing and educating the patient about the disease and its treatments can prevent treatment failure.

As the literature helps to elucidate the factors that affect the quality of life of patients with psoriasis, healthcare professionals can become more attuned to their delicate interplay and powerful consequences. Meaningful improvement in psoriasis necessitates awareness of the range of problems these patients face: the cutaneous manifestations including pain and pruritus, and the physical, psychosocial and economic impact the disease has on a patient's quality of life.

References

1 Rapp SR, Feldman SR, Exum ML, Fleischer AB Jr, Reboussin DM (1999) Psorasis causes as much disability as other major medical diseases. *J Am Acad Dermatol* 41: 401–407

2 Shumaker SA, Naughton MJ (1995) The international assessment of health-related quality of life. In: RA Shumaker, R Berzon (eds): *The international assessment of health-related quality of life theory, translation, measurement, and analysis*. Rapid Communications; New York, 3–10

3 NPF Survey Panel (2006) http://www.psoriasis.org/files/pdfs/research/2006_spring_survey_panel.pdf

4 Kirby B, Richards HL, Woo P, Hindle E, Main CJ, Griffiths CE (2001) Physical and psychologic measures are necessary to assess overall psoriasis severity. *J Am Acad Dermatol* 45(1): 72–76

5 Zachariae R, Zachariae H, Blomqvist K, Davidsson S, Molin L, Mork C, Sigurgeirsso B (2002) Epidemiology and Health Services Research: Quality of life in 6497 Nordic patients with psoriasis. *Br J Dermatol* 146: 1006–1016

6 Finlay AY, Ortonne JP (2004) Patient satisfaction with psoriasis therapies: an update and introduction to biologic therapy. *J Cut Med Surg* 8: 310–320

7 Mease PJ, Menter MA (2006) Quality-of-life issues in psoriasis and psoriatic arthritis: Outcome measures and therapies from a dermatological perspective. *J Am Acad Dermatol* 54: 685–704

8 Gordon K, Korman N, Frankel E, Wang H, Jahreis A, Zitnik R, Chang T (2006) Efficacy of etanercept in an integrated multistudy database of patients with psoriasis. *J Am Acad Dermatol* 54: S101–111

9 Fortune, DG, Richards HL, Griffiths CEM (2005) Pyschological factors in psoriasis: consequences, mechanisms, and interventions. *Dermatol Clin* 23: 681–694

10 Krueger G, Koo J, Lebwohl M, Menter A, Stern RS, Rolstad T (2001) The impact of psoriasis on quality of life: results of a 1998 National Psorasis Foundation patient-membership survey. *Arch Dermatol* 137: 280–284

11 NPF Survey Panel Fall (2005) http://www.psoriasis.org/files/pdfs/research/2005_fall_survey_panel.pdf

12 Dubertret L, Mrowietz U, Ranki A, van de Kerkhof PC, Chimenti S, Lotti T, Schafer G (2006) European patient perspectives on the impact of psoriasis: the EUROPSO patient membership survey. *Br J Dermatol* 155: 729–736

13 Yosipovitch G, Tang MBY (2000) Practical management of psoriasis in the elderly. *Drugs Aging* 19(11): 847–863

14 Gladman DD, Helliwell P, Mease PJ, Nash P, Ritchlin C, Taylor W (2004) Assessment of patients with psoriatic arthritis: a review of currently available measures. *Arthritis Rheum* 50: 24–35

15 De Jong EM, Seegers BA, Gulinck MK, Boezeman JB, van de Kerkhof PC (1996) Psoriasis of the nails associated with disability in a large number of patients: results of a recent interview with 1'728 patients. *Dermatology* 193: 300–303

16 Pettey AA, Balkrishnan R, Rapp SR, Fleischer AB, Feldman SR (2003) Patients with palmoplantar psoriasis have more physical disability and discomfort than patients with other forms of psoriasis: implications for clinical practice. *J Am Acad Dermatol* 49: 271–275

17 NPF Survey Panel Fall 2004: http://www.psoriasis.org/files/pdfs/research/2004_fall_survey_panel.pdf

18 Pearce DJ, Singh S, Balkrishnan R, Kulkarni A, Fleischer AB, Feldman SR (2006) The negative impact of psoriasis on the workplace. *J Dermatolog Treat* 17(1): 24–28

19 Finlay AY, Coles E (1995) The effect of severe psoriasis on the quality of life of 369 patients. *Br J Dermatol* 132: 236–244

20 Schmitt JM, Ford DE (2006) Work limitations and productivity loss are associated with health-related quality of life but not with clinical severity in patients with psoriasis. *Dermatology* 213(2): 102–110

21 Marchetti A, LaPensee K, An P (1998) A pharmacoeconomic analysis of topical therapies for

patients with mild-to-moderate stable plaque psoriasis: a US study. *Clinical Therapy* 20(4): 8518–8569
22 Esposito M, Saraceno R, Giunta A, Maccarone M, Chimenti S (2006) An Italian study on psoriasis and depression. *Dermatology* 212(2): 123–127
23 Picardi A, Abeni D, Melchi CF, Puddu P, Pasquini P (2000) Psychiatric morbidity in dermatological outpatients: an issue to be recognized. *Br J Dermatol* 143: 983–991
24 Gupta MA, Gupta AK (1998) Depression and suicidal ideation in dermatology patients with acne, alopecia areata, atopic dermatitis and psoriasis. *Br J Dermatol* 139: 846–850
25 Devrimci-Ozguven H, Kundakci TN, Kumbasar H, Boyvat A (2000) The depression, anxiety and life satisfaction and affective expression level in psoriasis patients. *J Eur Acad Deramtol Venereol* 14: 267–271
26 Gupta MA, Gupta AK (1999) Depression modulates pruritus perception: a study of pruritus in psoriasis, atopic dermatitis and chronic idiopathic urticaria. *Ann NY Acad Sci* 885: 394–395
27 Gupta MA, Gupta AK, Watteel GN (1998) Perceived deprivation of social touch in psoriasis associated with greater psychologic morbidity: an index of the stigma experience in dermatologic disorders. *Cutis* 61: 339–342
28 Richards HL, Fortune DG, Griffiths CE, Main CJ (2001) The contribution of perceptions of stigmatization to disability in patients with psoriasis. *J Psychosom Res* 50: 11–15
29 Fortune DG, Main CJ, O'Sullivan TM, Griffiths CE (1997) Quality of life in psoriasis: the contribution of clinical variables and psoriasis-specific stress. *Br J Dermatol* 137: 755–760
30 Fortune DG, Main CJ, O'Sullivan TM, Griffiths CE (1997) Assessing illness-related stress in psoriasis: the psychometric properties of the Psoriasis Life Stress Inventory. *J Psychosom Res* 42: 467–476
31 Fortune DG, Richards HL, Kirby B, McElhone K, Markham T, Rogers S, Main CJ, Griffiths CE (2003) Psychological distress impairs clearance of psoriasis in patients treated with photochemotherapy. *Arch Dermatol* 139: 752–756
32 Vardy D, Besser A, Amir M, Gesthalter B, Biton A, Buskila D (2002) Experiences of stigmatization play a role in mediating the impact of disease severity on quality of life in psoriasis patients. *Br J Dermatol* 147: 736–742
33 33Sampogna F, Picardi A, Melchi CF, Pasquini P, Abeni D (2003) The impact of skin diseases on patients: comparing dermatologists' opinions with research data collected on their patients. *Br J Dermatol* 148: 989–995
34 Gupta MA, Gupta AK (1995) Age and gender differences in the impact of psoriasis on quality of life. *Int J Dermatol* 34: 700–703
35 Sampogna F, Chren MM, Melchi CF, Pasquini P, Tabolli S, Abeni D (2006) Age, gender, quality of life and psychological distress in patients hospitalized with psoriasis. *Br J Dermatol* 154: 325–331
36 Zachariae R, Zachariae C, Ibsen H, Mortensen JT, Wulf HC (2000) Dermatology life quality index: data from Danish inpatients and outpatients. *Acta Derm Venereol* 80: 272–276
37 Schmid-Ott G, Kunsebeck HW, Jager B, Sittig U, Hofste N, Ott R, Malewski P, Lamprecht F (2005) Significance of the stigmatization experience of psoriasis patients: a 1-year follow-up of the illness and its psychosocial consequences in men and women. *Acta Derm Venereol* 85(1): 27–32
38 Ginsburg IH (1996) The psychosocial impact of skin disease. *Dermatol Clin* 14: 473–484
39 Koo J (1996) Population-based epidemiologic study of psoriasis with emphasis on quality of life assessment. *Psychodermatology* 14: 485–496
40 Wahl A, Moum T, Hanestad BR, Wiklund I (1999) The relationship between demographic and clinical variables and quality of life aspects in patients with psoriasis. *Qual Life Res* 8: 319–326
41 Higgins E (2000) Alcohol, smoking and psoriasis. *Clin Exp Dermatol* 25: 108–110
42 Unaeze J, Nijsten T, Murphy A, Ravichandran C, Stern RS (2006) Impact of psoriasis on health-related quality of life decreases over time: an 11-year prospective study. *J Invest Dermatol* 126: 1480–1489
43 Ellis CN, Mordin MM, Adler EY (2003) Effects of Alefacept on health-related quality of life in patients with psoriasis: results from a randomized, placebo-controlled phase II trial. *Am J Clin Dermatol* 4: 131–139
44 Krueger GG, Langley RG, Finlay AY, Griffiths CE, Woolley JM, Lalla D, Jahreis A (2005) Patient-reported outcomes of psoriasis improvement with etanercept therapy: results of a randomized phase III trial. *Br J Dermatol* 153: 1192–1199

45 Gordon K, Korman N, Frankel E, Wang H, Jahreis A, Zitnik R, Chang T (2006) Efficacy of etanercept in an integrated multistudy database of patients with psoriasis. *J Am Acad Dermatol* 54: S101–111
46 Krueger G, Wooley JM, Zitnik R (2004) The effects of etanercept therapy on patient reported outcomes for patients with moderate to severe psoriasis. Presented at the 62nd annual meeting of The American Academy of Dermatology, 6–11 Feb 2004, Washington D.C.
47 Leonardi CL, Powers JL, Matheson RT, Goffe BS, Zitnik R, Wang A, Gottlieb AB (2003) Etanercept as monotherapy in patients with psoriasis. *N Engl J Med* 349: 2014–2022
48 Feldman SR, Kimball AB, Krueger GG, Woolley JM, Lalla D, Jahreis A (2005) Etanercept improves the health-related quality of life of patients with psoriasis: results of a phase III randomized clinical trial. *J Am Acad Dermatol* 53(5): 887–889
49 Feldman SR, Menter A, Koo JY (2004) Improved health-related quality of life following a randomized controlled trial of alefacept treatment in patients with chronic plaque psoriasis. *Br J Dermatol* 150: 317–326
50 Ortonne J, Shear N, Shumack S, Henninger E (2005) Impact of efalizumab on patient-reported outcomes in high-need psoriasis patients: results of the international, randomized, placebo-controlled Phase III Clinical Experience Acquired with Raptiva (CLEAR) trial [NCT00256139]. *BMC Dermatology* 5: 13
51 Koo JY, Kowalksi J, Guenther L, Walker P (2004) Quality of life effect of oral tazarotene in patients with moderate to severe psoriasis as measured by the 12-item psoriasis quality of life questionnaire (PQOL-12). Presented at the 62nd annual meeting of the American Academy of Dermatology; 6–11 Feb 2004, Washington D.C.
52 Lim C, Brown P (2006) Quality of life in psoriasis improves after standardized administration of narrowband UVB phototherapy. *Australas J Dermatol* 47(1): 37–40
53 Kaltwasser JP, Nash P, Gladman D, Rosen CF, Behrens F, Jones P, Wollenhaupt J, Falk FG, Mease P (2004) Efficacy and safety of leflunomide in the treatment of psoriatic arthritis and psoriasis: a multinational, double-blind, randomized, placebo-controlled clinical trial. *Arthritis Rheum* 50: 1939–1950
54 Salek MS, Finlay AY, Lewis JJ, Sumner MI (2004) Quality of life and clinical outcome in psoriasis patients using intermittent cyclosporin (Neoral.) *Qual Life Res* 13: 91–95
55 Bhosle MJ, Kulkarni A, Feldman S, Balkrishnan R (2006) Quality of life in patients with psoriasis. *Health and Quality of Life Outcomes* 4: 35
56 Heydendael VM, Spuls PI, Opmeer BC, de Borgie CA, Reitsma JB, Goldschmidt WF, Bossuyt PM, Bos JD, de Rie MA (2003) Methotrexate *versus* cyclosporin in moderate-to-severe chronic plaque psoriasis. *N Engl J Med* 349: 658–665
57 Gottlieb AB, Ford RO, Spellman MC (2003) The efficacy and tolerability of clobetasol proprionate foam 0.05% in the treatment of mild to moderate plaque type psoriasis in nonscalp regions. J Cutan Med Surg 7: 185–*192*
58 Gupta MA, Gupta AK (2001) The use of antidepressant drugs in dermatology. *J Eur Acad Dermatol Venereol* 15: 512–518
59 Zaghloul SS, Goodfield MJ (2004) Objective Assessment of compliance with psoriasis treatment. *Arch Dermatol* 104: 408–414
60 David SE, Ahmed Z, Salek MS, Finlay AY (2005) Does enough quality of life-related discussion occur during dermatology outpatient consultations? *Br J Dermatol* 153: 997–1000
61 Feldman S, Behnam S, Behnam S, Koo JY (2005) Involving the patient: Impact of inflammatory skin disease and patient-focused care. *J Am Acad Dermatol* 53: S78–85
62 Lu Y, Duller P, van der Valk PGM, Kraaimaat FW, van de Kerkhof PC (2003) Helplessness as predictor of perceived stigmatization in patients with psoriasis and atopic dermatitis. *Dermatol Psychosom* 4: 146–150
63 de Korte J, van Onselen J, Kownacki S (2005) Quality of care in patients with psoriasis: an initial clinical study of an international disease management programme. *J EurAcad Dermatol Venereol* 19(1): 35–41
64 NPF website, http://www.psoriasis.org/advocacy/
65 Gordon K (2005) Patient education and advocacy Groups. *Arch Dermatol* (141): 80–81
66 Nijsten T, Rolstad T, Feldman SR, Stern RS (2005) Members of the National Psoriasis Foundation: more extensive disease and better informed about treatment options. *Arch Dermatol* 141: 19–26
67 Jankowiak B, Krajewska-Kulak E, Baranowska A (2005) The importance of the health education

in life quality improvement in patients with psoriasis. *Rocz Akad Med Bialmyst* 50 Suppl 1: 145–147
68 Fortune DG, Richards HL, Main CJ, Bowcock S, Main CJ, Griffiths CE (2002) A cognitive-behavioural symptom management programme as an adjunct in psoriasis therapy. *Br J Dermatol* 146: 458–465
69 Price, ML, Mottahedin I, Mayo PR (1991) Can psychotherapy help patients with psoriasis? *Clin Exp Dermatol* 16(2): 114–117
70 Kabat-Zinn J, Wheeler E, Light T, Skillings A, Scharf M, Cropley T, Hosmer D, Bernhard J (1998) Influence of a mindfulness meditation-based stress reduction intervention on rates of skin clearing in patients with moderate to severe psoriasis undergong phototherapy (UVB) and photochemotherapy (PUVA). *Psychosomatic Med* 60: 625–632
71 Koblenzer CS (1987) *Psychocutaneous disease.* Grune and Stratton, Orlando, Florida, US
72 Britten N, Stevenson FA, Barry CA, Barber N, Bradley CP (2000) Misunderstandings in prescribing decisions in general practice: qualitative study. *BMJ* 320: 484–488

Index

The MDT-Series
Milestones in Drug Therapy

The discovery of drugs is still an unpredictable process. Breakthroughs are often the result of a combination of factors, including serendipidity, rational strategies and a few individuals with novel ideas. *Milestones in Drug Therapy* highlights new therapeutic developments that have provided significant steps forward in the fight against disease. Each book deals with an individual drug or drug class that has altered the approach to therapy. Emphasis is placed on the scientific background to the discoveries and the development of the therapy, with an overview of the current state of knowledge provided by experts in the field, revealing also the personal stories behind these milestone developments. The series is aimed at a broad readership, covering biotechnology, biochemistry, pharmacology and clinical therapy.

Forthcoming titles

Echinocandin Antifungals, K. Bartizal, E. Hickey (Editors), 2008
Bipolar Depression: Molecular Neurobiology, Clinical Diagnosis and Pharmacotherapy, C.A. Zarate, H.K. Manji (Editors), 2008

Published volumes

Pharmacotherapy of Obesity, J.P.H. Wilding (Editor), 2008
Entry Inhibitors in HIV Therapy, J.D. Reeves, C.A. Derdeyn (Editors), 2007
Drugs affecting Growth of Tumours, H.M. Pinedo, C. Smorenburg (Editors), 2006
TNF-alpha Inhibitors, J.M. Weinberg, R. Buchholz (Editors), 2006
Aromatase Inhibitors, B.J.A. Furr (Editor), 2006
Cannabinoids as Therapeutics, R. Mechoulam (Editor), 2005
St. John's Wort and its Active Principles in Anxiety and Depression, W.E. Müller (Editor), 2005
Drugs for Relapse Prevention of Alcoholism, R. Spanagel, K. Mann (Editors), 2005
COX-2 Inhibitors, M. Pairet, J. Van Ryn (Editors), 2004
Calcium Channel Blockers, T. Godfraind (Author), 2004
Sildenafil, U. Dunzendorfer (Editor), 2004
Hepatitis Prevention and Treatment, J. Colacino, B.A. Heinz (Editors), 2004
Combination Therapy of AIDS, E. De Clercq, A.M. Vandamme (Editors), 2004
Cognitive Enhancing Drugs, J. Buccafusco (Editor), 2004
Fluoroquinolone Antibiotics, A.R. Ronald, D. Low (Editors), 2003

Erythropoietins and Erythropoiesis, G. Molineux, M. Foote, S. Elliott (Editors), 2003
Macrolide Antibiotics, W. Schönfeld, H. Kirst (Editors), 2002
HMG CoA Reduktase Inhibitors, G. Schmitz, M. Torzewski (Editors), 2002
Antidepressants, B.E. Leonard (Editor), 2001
Recombinant Protein Drugs, P. Buckel (Editor), 2001
Glucocorticoids, N. Goulding, R.J. Flower (Editors), 2001
Modern Immunosuppressives, H.-J. Schuurman (Editor), 2001
ACE Inhibitors, P. D'Orleans-Juste, G. Plante (Editors), 2001
Atypical Antipsychotics, A.R. Cools, B.A. Ellenbroek (Editors), 2000
Methotrexate, B.N. Cronstein, J.R. Bertino (Editors), 2000
Anxiolytics, M. Briley, D. Nutt (Editors), 2000
Proton Pump Inhibitors, L. Olbe (Editor), 1999
Valproate, W. Löscher (Editor), 1999